# THE ONE-TEN-TEN METHOD FOR ALLERGY CONTROL

*The One-Ten-Ten Method for Allergy Control* is a self-help program based upon the principle that allergy symptoms are related in part to psychological stress. While a great deal of attention has been given to the physical and chemical nature of allergy, the psychological factors largely have been ignored. The One-Ten-Ten Method confronts this issue squarely and shows how to bring the symptoms of wheezing, sneezing, and coughing under the control of one's own will through the process of autosuggestion and self-imaging.

The scientific basis of The One-Ten-Ten Method is well documented. Allergy symptoms are known to be triggered by that portion of the brain called *hypothalamus*. The ten simple mental exercises outlined in this book were developed by the author—himself an allergy victim of the worst magnitude—as a means of relaxing the brain and re-programming the hypothalamus. Anyone can do it—even children!

The One-Ten-Ten Method is, by its very nature, a non-drug approach to allergy control. It can be used as an alternative or supplement to conventional treatment.

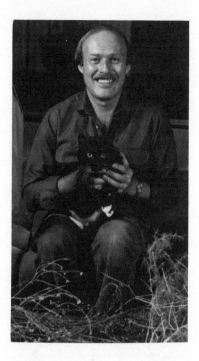

## *John A. Laccinole*

John A. Laccinole is a business executive residing in Southern California with his wife, Mary, and their two children, Christine and Kathleen. He holds a Masters degree in Business Administration. His research in the area of allergy control was a result of concern about his own illness. Diagnosed as having severe hay fever (perennial allergic diathesis with vasomotor rhinitis) and with early symptoms of emphysema, Mr. Laccinole tried all of the standard drug-related therapies to no avail. In desperation he turned to the medical literature and discovered several obscure references to the relationship between allergy symptoms and malfunction of the hypothalamus region of the brain. Coupling this information with certain techniques of autosuggestion that were developed as part of an executive motivational program utilized by his company, he synthesized an entirely new approach to the treatment of allergies—*and it worked!* Initially,  all the experimentation with the One-Ten-Ten Method was conducted on himself. After perfecting the technique through trial and error, however, he began to share his discovery with other allergy sufferers. News of each success spread like wildfire, and soon the demand for photocopies of his notes and instructions became so great that he was forced to seek a publisher to organize and distribute his program in the form of a book. This volume is the result of that effort.

# THE
# ONE-TEN-TEN METHOD
# FOR ALLERGY CONTROL

A Non-drug Approach
for the Relief of
Hay Fever and Bronchial Asthma

by John A. Laccinole

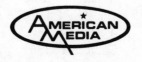

American Media
790 Hampshire Rd., Suite H
Westlake Village,
California 91361

This book is dedicated to the world's untold millions who suffer from allergies.

It is also dedicated to their unfortunate friends and families who have been compelled to share their affliction by association.

May The One-Ten-Ten Method bring them the joy of a rich and normal life once again.

I would like to express my deepest appreciation to the many friends and associates who helped make this book possible; especially to my wife, Mary, and my daughters, Christine, and Kathleen for their endless patience and understanding during the dark years; to H. James Zinger for his kind introduction to this book and for first introducing me to the autosuggestion techniques that became the core of The One-Ten-Ten Method; to Dr. Walter Siporin for his personal encouragement to continue with my experiments in the early stages of development; to G. Edward Griffin for editing my manuscript and for his excellent two-chapter contribution in the Publisher's Supplement; to Glenora Palumbo, William Pyestner, Patricia Griffin, Rhonda and Wally Jukes, Maria de la Luz Monarrez, and Len Mazzuca, for their valuable help and cooperation at every step along the way.

*John A. Laccinole*

# CONTENTS

An introduction to The One-Ten-Ten Method; a definition of primary
terms; a review of allergy symptoms; the importance of emotional factors
and their impact on the hypothalamus region of the brain.

A review of the author's own ten-year battle against the symptoms of
allergy: the first attack at age thirty; unsuccessful attempts to avoid
allergy-producing elements; decline in health; eight years of dependence on desensitizing shots; agony and frustration resulting from only
partial control and frequent relapses prior to The One-Ten-Ten Method.

The author takes a hard look in retrospect at the emotional factors that
were present in his own life and suggests that these, not only were pivotal
in bringing on his own attacks, but may be fairly representative of similar
factors found in the lives of many allergy sufferers.

A review of the background events and rationale that culminated in the
creation of The One-Ten-Ten Method; initial experience with the
method; decision to publish.

Step-by-step instructions on how to prepare oneself for successfully
applying the method; selecting the right location; how to relax; how to
breathe; specific phrases to be committed to memory. This is the core of
the self-imaging program.

# FOREWORD

By H. James Zinger
President,
Hypmovation Inc.

For over twenty years, I have been a professional in the field of hypnosis, helping people to improve the quality of their businesses, their families, and their personal lives. In that period of time, I have worked with two medical clinics which utilized hypnotic techniques for changing attitudes, habits, and behavior. I have come across thousands of people who have suffered from allergies, and many of them have experienced substantial relief or, in some cases, complete alleviation of all symptoms through utilizing techniques that are similar to the One-Ten-Ten Method.

Over the years, I have endeavored to search out books on methods of mind control over allergies. To the best of my knowledge, there are none that hit the subject as directly and positively as does Mr. Laccinole's present volume. The content is easy to understand and comes directly to the point. It covers only the areas of importance and it gives specific techniques for making the program work.

I have found from my own personal experiences with allergies that a great deal of the problem is psychological. Most individuals who suffer from allergies or hay fever tend to surround themselves with others who have similar problems so they can commiserate with each other about the agony of sneezing, coughing, congestion, runny and itchy eyes, and all of the other problems that they share. This reaffirms the negative aspect of their affliction and causes them to lock in psychologically, to imprint upon the hopelessness of their situation, all of which only serves to aggravate the allergy and make it worse.

The conscious mind represents only about ten per cent of our total mental capacity. That is the part of the mind we use when we dwell upon our problems. If we hold negative thoughts in our minds long enough, we actually can create the very things we dread the most. The conscious mind, however, does not remember. The *subconscious* is the storehouse of everything we have ever heard, seen, felt, smelled, touched, or experienced since the day we were born. It is this vast subconscious mind that also keeps us following certain behavior patterns. Even though allergy victims might *consciously* want to change their attitudes, the *subconscious* mind can be like a magnet pulling them back into negative thinking. Every time they sneeze, they think, "Is the pollen heavy? Is this happening again?" and they actually start to hypnotize themselves into the negative feelings, the emotions, the total experience of hay fever.

It has been estimated that eighty-seven per cent of all illnesses are psychosomatic, or in the mind. That certainly includes allergies and the symptoms of allergies. The nervous system does not know the difference between real experiences and imagined experiences. This is why, when people start thinking about pollens, they can develop the symptoms of allergy whether there are pollens in the air or not. They find themselves going through all of the physical trauma even though the problem is caused psychologically. The One-Ten-Ten Method, therefore, is an excellent procedure for reversing this cycle by re-programming the thinking processes. Getting people to think of the end result, of the way they want to breathe and how they want to feel is the main objective, and it should definitely put anyone onto the right track.

Many people, when they have allergies in certain seasons, are told by their doctors to change their environment, to get away from the area in which they live, or the trees, shrubs, or flowers that surround them. No one is talking about changing the *psychological* environment, and that is one of the most important things. When an athlete becomes proficient at his sport, most people do not realize that his psychological conditioning is as important, if not more so, than his physical conditioning. Mr. Laccinole has applied this reality to the study of health. His book stands alone in its field. It is the only one that teaches people how to deal psychologically with allergies. It represents a giant step forward in the alleviation of one of man's most baffling diseases.

# I

# BASICS FIRST

*An introduction to The One-Ten-Ten
Method; a definition of primary
terms; a review of allergy symptoms; the importance of emotional
factors and their impact on the
hypothalamus region of the brain.*

Man basically is a creature of habit. Occasionally, it
becomes necessary to alter those habits or to replace
them with new ones. The purpose of The One-Ten-Ten
Method is to give the reader the ability to form new
mental habits. After the method is mastered, it will
enable an individual to program the subconscious mind
which, in turn, will control the symptoms associated
with allergies, especially hay fever (allergic rhinitis) and
bronchial asthma.

The One-Ten-Ten Method is a subconscious development technique utilizing words and phrases as
subconscious implants. The method uses an individual's own mental energy for the control and relief of
allergy symptoms. It is an alternative or supplement to
conventional treatment.

**A Subconscious
Technique**

Before delving into The One-Ten-Ten Method itself,
it is imperative that we have a basic understanding of
allergies, their causes, their symptoms, and the traditional treatment.

**35,000,000 sufferers**    In the United States alone, it is estimated that thirty-five million people suffer from allergies. Approximately nine million of these have been diagnosed as suffering from asthma. This can be considered as nothing less than an epidemic.

An allergy can develop at any age, even during infancy. It is not uncommon for a person in the middle years of life suddenly to experience a first allergy attack. No age group or race or sex is immune.

The basic definition of the word allergy, according to Webster's Encyclopedic Dictionary, is an excess sensitivity to substances, such as pollen, food, drugs, heat, or cold, which are harmless to most persons. Common allergy reactions are hay fever, hives, and bronchial asthma.

**Hay fever**    The disease originally was called *hay fever* in England because it was most prevalent during the haying season. We now know that hay is not the only cause of hay fever.

The medical name for hay fever is *allergic rhinitis*. It also has been called allergic coryza, rose fever, pollinosis, summer catarrh, and vasomotor rhinitis.

The symptoms of a hay fever attack are generally well known. The most obvious ones are red eyes, itching and runny nose, and attacks of explosive sneezing. In advanced cases, there is a serious complication that can occur when the sensitivity extends into the mucous membranes of the lungs. This can produce symptoms of wheezing, difficulty in breathing, and an annoying cough. If untreated, this condition generally progresses

**Bronchial asthma**    into *bronchial asthma*.

Bronchial asthma is an allergy with sensitivity in the lungs and bronchial passages. The clinical symptoms are wheezing and shortness of breath. The chain of events leading up to an asthmatic attack are similar to those that trigger a hay fever attack. Common offending substances as they are breathed through the nose, are pollens of trees, shrubs, grasses, and flowers, as well as dander, house dust, and certain chemicals.

In both asthma and hay fever, these irritants cause the body to produce histamine which, in turn, causes the symptoms of allergy. In the nose, histamine induces profuse secretion of mucus. In the bronchial passages, histamine causes a reduced ability to breathe and other symptoms associated with bronchial asthma. The treatment for both hay fever and asthma generally is the same.

**Histamine**

The diagnosis of allergy is made by a physician on the basis of symptoms, hereditary background, and tests. The most common test is the skin test in which pollen or other suspected irritants are introduced into the skin through a scratch.

The most common form of treatment today is the injection of pollen or other specific irritants to "desensitize" the patient. Most allergists advocate the use of antihistamines, as needed, in addition to the injections.

Many scientists now believe that allergy is psychogenic in origin. It has been proven that, under psychological stimulation, hay fever symptoms can be reproduced. Mental suggestion has been used in select cases as a method of controlling hay fever attacks. When considering the treatment of allergy, it is essential to take into consideration the emotional factor as well as the physical nature of the condition. In allergy, as in other diseases, the psychological factors constitute a force that can upset the normal equilibrium of the body.

**The psychological factor**

As an example of the way our emotions can effect the symptoms of allergy, many physicians have found that people can bring on an attack of sneezing, wheezing, nasal blockage, or rash simply by experiencing fear, stress, or anguish. Symptoms can be produced solely by emotional trauma.

There is a region in the brain called the *hypothalamus*. Acting like a computer, the hypothalamus regulates the activities associated with the autonomic nervous system.

**The hypothalamus**

We cannot consciously control its activities but, nevertheless, its function can be altered by our emotional state. The extent to which we can control our emotional state is the extent to which we can effect the hypothalamus. Its function, therefore, is partially within our control.

For reasons that are not fully understood, the bodily functions normally regulated automatically by the hypothalamus are the same ones that are involved in allergy reactions. For example, asthmatic or hay fever sufferers may find that their breathing no longer is automatically adjusted to meet their need. This inability to breathe normally often creates a panic-fear reaction, which is understandable. This condition of fright, however, often causes the symptoms to get worse, leading to more fear, and so forth.

**Panic-fear syndrome**

The autonomic nervous system is connected with areas in the brain involved with both thought and feeling. The presence of problems or worries in our subconscious mind can have an effect on the hypothalamus, and, in this way, may help to bring on an allergy attack.

---

For a more detailed analysis of the technical aspects of how The One-Ten-Ten Method works, with particular emphasis on the involvement of the hypothalamus, the pituitary gland, and the autonomic nervous system, I strongly recommend that you turn to the Publisher's Supplement in the back of this book and read G. Edward Griffin's excellent chapter entitled *It's Dynamite.* If you are *not* interested in the scientific basis behind The One-Ten-Ten Method, then you may wish to skip over that material and continue directly to Chapter Two.

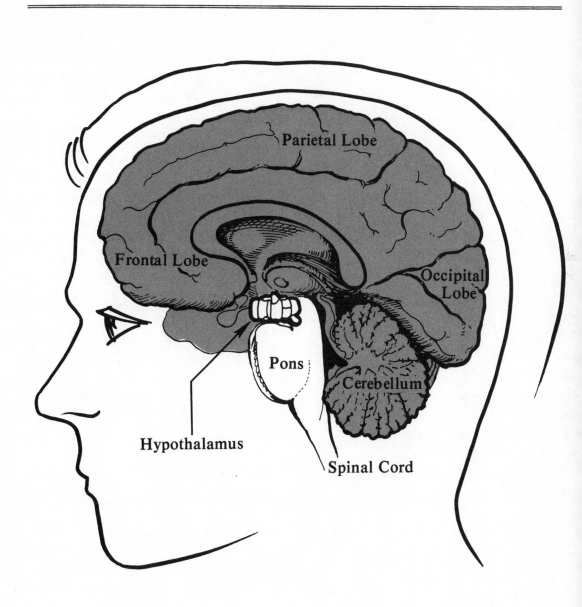

*Hypothalamus nestled in center of brain*

# II

# A TYPICAL MEDICAL HISTORY

*A review of the author's own ten-year battle against the symptoms of allergy: the first attack at age thirty; unsuccessful attempts to avoid allergy – producing elements; decline in health; eight years of dependence on desensitizing shots; agony and frustration resulting from only partial control and frequent relapses prior to The One-Ten-Ten Method.*

In order to have a more clear understanding of The One-Ten-Ten Method and its development, it will be helpful for you to know something of my own ten-year battle against allergies, for this is the background of desperation that generated the motivation to seek alternative therapies and to experiment in the creation of new ones.

**How it all began**

My first allergy attacks began in the latter months of 1969. At first, I thought merely that I had a persistent cold and did not relate my sneezing, wheezing, running eyes, running nose, and coughing to allergy. But as the weeks slipped by and the year drew to a close, the symptoms refused to leave. I was thirty years old at the time and became distressed that, at my age, I couldn't seem to throw a simple cold.

By 1970, I had become truly desperate. All of my symptoms continued, and the attacks became more frequent and more severe. Friends began to suggest that I might have had "hay fever," and freely offered advice on how to treat it. I can remember the suggestions quite vividly.

Someone suggested that I was allergic to trees, shrubs, and other assorted vegetation surrounding my home. I immediately set out to rectify the situation. I uprooted the shrubs, down went the trees, out went the plants—but to no avail. My nose continued to run, unabated, day and night.

It was suggested that I give up certain beverages such as beer and wine on the remote possibility that one or both were serving as a trigger for my attacks. I totally discontinued any consumption of these beverages for several months in order to give this possibility total benefit of the doubt. The theory proved unfounded. I continued, as before, sneezing, wheezing, and coughing.

During this period, it also was suggested that our household pets might be the culprits and that they should be given away. Needless to say, this proposal was not kindly received by my wife and daughters. The idea was shelved temporarily in hopes that some other more "humane" solution could be found.

As the year 1970 progressed, my allergy attacks increased in frequency until they were almost non-stop. My nose literally was running twenty-four hours a day. It looked like a red warning beacon in the snow. Friends **Rudolph the** began to make jokes about Rudolph the Red-nosed **Red-nosed Reindeer** Reindeer. I laughed, but, to me, it wasn't very funny.

By mid-1970, my affliction began to affect, not only my physical health, but my mental well-being as well. My personal relationships to family, friends, and fellow workers began to deteriorate badly. I lost my temper easily and was in a constant state of irritability. I believe this was caused by chronic lack of sleep. It was routine for me to awaken in the middle of the night, coughing and sneezing, and then be unable to return to sleep without taking an antihistamine. Once I took a shot of cortisone to see if that would stop the drainage. It did not help. At one point during a particularly severe attack, I actually sniffed ammonia fumes in a desperate attempt to cauterize my nose. It didn't work, of course, and I quickly regretted the attempt. Between this pill and that, I became a walking medicine chest, and it is possible that the constant intake of drugs also was a contributing factor to my decline in physical and mental health.

**A walking medicine chest**

Finally, in September of 1970, I decided to seek professional medical help. During my initial visit with the allergist, I was told there was an excellent possibility that I had allergies. (I knew *that* already. That's why I had come to him in the first place!) The doctor scheduled me for testing to determine what type of plants, animals, or substances might be the cause of my problem. The tests revealed that I was allergic to just about everything that grows or walks on four legs. Not only was I allergic to cats, dogs, camels, feather pillows, kapok, and goats, but also to the all-time classic mugwort. That's right, friends, MUGWORT!

**Allergic to almost everything**

After I digested all of this good news, I began a series of injections that would continue through two doctors and last until April 15, 1979—a total period of about eight-and-a-half years. The purpose of these shots was to "desensitize" me. With the process of desensitization under way (which consisted of bi-weekly and then weekly injections), I found time to discuss the possible causes of my condition with my doctor. Several interesting medical views were brought into focus during the conversations:

**Desensitizing shots**

1. Allergies can be inherited.
2. Allergies are classified as a disease.
3. The only way one can get total relief from allergies is to move to Nome, Alaska, and live in an igloo.

**Medical viewpoint, 1970**

4. Allergies can occur at any age.
5. Relief and control can be obtained through desensitization shots.

This was the medical viewpoint as explained to me in 1970.

The desensitization process did help relieve some of the symptoms associated with my allergy. Severe attacks were still a very real part of my life, but they became less frequent and of shorter duration than those I had experienced previously. I also was taking antihistamines on a daily basis which helped to relieve the sneezing and nose flow. I was still a walking pharmacy and my health suffered from that fact, but I was grateful for whatever relief I could get.

In 1971, we moved from a home located near the beach in Los Angeles to a spot several miles inland: the San Fernando Valley. Temperatures were higher, and the absence of an ocean breeze made me aware more than ever before of all the things that grow and live on land. I changed allergists in 1973 and had myself re-tested. There was no change in my areas of sensitivity with the exception of oak trees. My sensitivity to oak trees actually had *increased* instead of decreased with the desensitizing injections.

**Getting worse, not better**

At first, I received injections twice a week. As time progressed, however, they were administered once a week, then once every two weeks, and then once every three weeks.

**A very serious mistake**

Soon after reaching the three-week level, I decided to stop my injections, because I thought I was cured. Well, I quit and nearly *died.* Several weeks after my injection was due, I had a full-blown allergy attack which put me in bed for a week. The attack included a continuous fever, running nose, coughing, and sneezing. One eye actually closed for several days because of the swelling. Needless to say, I immediately went back on the needle. My desensitization continued until April 15, 1979. By that time, I had graduated to only one shot per month.

As I have mentioned previously, the desensitization process was a tremendous help, but it did have questionable side-effects and it did not control my symptoms completely. Perhaps I can best illustrate this by relating several occurrences that took place at various intervals over the years.

Before I became somewhat of a conservationist, I was an occasional bird hunter. Every year I would go dove or pheasant hunting and enjoy myself immensely walking through the fields. I can vividly recall the last time I went hunting. I was in an open field when the attack hit me. From that instant forward, the birds were in no danger. Not only were they given ample warning by my loud nasal explosions, but there was no chance in the world that I would *accurately* squeeze off a shot while sneezing, coughing, choking, and wiping my nose! My days as the great game bird hunter had come to an end.

**Goodby bird hunting**

One of the most aggravating things for me to accept was not being able to work in my yard, particularly during the spring and autumn months. The only way to avoid an attack during these seasons was to load up with antihistamines before stepping out the door. Being an outdoors person, I found this situation extremely frustrating.

My allergies also proved to be a serious handicap in the performance of my job. In management, one occasionally must conduct meetings for communications or for training personnel. On many such occasions I would have a sudden allergy attack and have to leave the room right in the middle of the meeting. To say the least, this is not the path to rapid advancement in one's work.

**A handicap on the job**

Driving a car during an attack is, of course, a monumental challenge. Most of you who are reading these pages are quite familiar with the problem. You *know* what it is like to be caught in rush hour traffic—

**A menace on the road**

bumper to bumper—and suddenly be overcome with a four-star attack. Your eyes start to water and you can't see. You sneeze all over your windshield. You begin choking. The attack goes on and on and on, and you *can't* pull off to the side! It's a wonder that any of us are still alive to talk about it.

It is impossible to recount all of the problems created by my affliction over the years. But it is not necessary, for yours are probably much the same as mine. The reason I have subjected you to my personal story merely is to let you know that I have come to this subject from *experience*. My discovery was born, not of academic interest, but of necessity and desperation.

After I had developed The One-Ten-Ten Method and found myself in control of my allergy, I was able to go back in memory and to construct a personal profile of psychological factors that may have contributed to my condition. The next chapter deals with that profile.

# III

# THE LIVE OAKS INCIDENT

*The author takes a hard look in retrospect at the emotional factors that were present in his own life and suggests that these, not only were pivotal in bringing on his own attacks, but may be fairly representative of similar factors found in the lives of many allergy sufferers.*

It was the spring of 1980. Pollen was in the air everywhere. Yet, it had been many months since I had my last allergy attack. As I sat at my desk effortlessly breathing the clean, fresh air wafting through the open window from the nearby fields, it was hard to turn my mind back to the "bad old days." As I forced myself to recall the details, however, a pattern began to emerge, and I couldn't help but wonder if it might have had something to do with my allergy. It was a pattern of stress.

This was my psychological profile:
1. During my formative childhood years, my mother was a hypochondriac, of sorts. She also suffers from allergies.
2. I lived with continual stress during my four years in the U.S. Marine Corps.

**A psychological profile**

3. I took on the responsibility of supporting a wife and children in my early twenties.
4. I went into management in 1967 and assumed responsibility for the success of others.
5. I purchased my second home in late 1970. At that time, I made what was considered to be a large financial commitment.
6. I quit smoking for the first time in 1969. It was during the latter part of 1969 that I experienced my first allergy attack.

**Anticipation of shots**

During the years of desensitization shots, 1970 to 1979, several personality changes occurred. One of the first things I noticed was that I developed an anticipation for my shot. I started talking about it several days in advance, and after I had my shot I actually became ill. I became depressed, dizzy, crabby, self-centered, and nauseous. It usually took about three days before these symptoms dissipated and allowed me to function again in a normal manner. The point, however, is that, in addition to the undesirable impact upon my personality and mood, I developed what appeared to be a strong psychological need for the shot, the symptoms, or both.

Looking back over my own performance, it is difficult to avoid the conclusion that I staged my attacks for the most opportune time to get what I wanted. Whenever I was around sympathetic people, and especially if I also was in a stressful situation, my eyes would water profusely, my upper lip would swell, and my nose would run like a faucet. I could always produce twenty to thirty whopping sneezes to cap off the performance. My **Benefits of an attack** reward for all of this was two-fold: (1) I received a great deal of attention and sympathy, and (2) my stress was partially relieved due to the implication that I wasn't really responsible for my obligations because of my obvious disability.

Perhaps the best way to illustrate how emotional

factors related to my own allergy is to tell you about a particularly severe attack that occurred several years before The One-Ten-Ten Method was developed. I call it "The Live Oaks Incident."

I was scheduled by my company to attend a management seminar in Fallbrook, California. I wasn't pleased about having to go and immediately developed a negative outlook. I tried to think of some way to avoid the affair, but attendance was absolutely required. I resented that almost as much as the seminar itself.

**A dreaded seminar**

When I told my family that I would be gone for a few days and that I would be housed in Fallbrook, my wife made plans for her and the children to meet me in Fallbrook at the conclusion of the seminar and then drive to the San Diego Wild Animal Park, which was not too far away. The plan then called for driving to the mountains for a few days to visit relatives in a place called Live Oaks.

**And worse to follow**

The whole thing sounded terrible from start to finish. First of all, I did not want to attend the seminar. Secondly, I knew that I would be tired and irritable after several days in meetings. I would not be ready to ride in a car full of kids, and definitely was not interested in the Wild Animal Park or Live Oaks. I rapidly built a solid negative wall of thought against the entire week. I *knew* I was going to have a terrible time.

Here is the sequence that followed. I complained daily for several weeks about having to attend the management seminar. When I actually got there, I was determined to prove that I had been right about not wanting to go. My attitude was characterized by such statements as "What a waste of time!" "I don't *believe* this!" and "They could have printed all this on a square of toilet paper!"

**A negative attitude**

When my family arrived to pick me up several days later, I was right on schedule. I promptly informed them that I had had a terrible time and that I was very, very tired.

The ride in the family car was not a disappointment. I hated it. By the time we got to the Wild Animal Park, I was ready to give the primal scream. The presence of animals gave me my cue and I began to sneeze. A massive sinus headache grabbed hold of my brain.

Upon arrival at Live Oaks, I was ready. All of the ingredients for an attack were there: sympathetic people, attention, and a huge oak tree growing directly over the house. Needless to say, I proceeded to stage the grand-daddy of all allergy attacks. I was literally flat on my back for the entire weekend, wheezing, sneezing, coughing, and blowing the old bugle. I was the center of attention and I had proven conclusively that I had been right about not wanting to go to the seminar, the zoo, and especially to Live Oaks. It was glorious.

**The granddaddy of all attacks**

After reading this, you may form the impression that my allergies were a kind of mental crutch. In my own case that is probably correct, although, I certainly didn't realize it at the time. I truly suffered, but there were definite side-advantages to my misery. I shall never really know to what extent my subconscious mind had come to anticipate and depend upon these subtle rewards.

I'm sure that this does *not* apply to all allergy sufferers, and, even in those cases where it does apply, it does not mean that the condition is faked. There is no one who has experienced such crippling attacks who willingly or knowingly would undergo one in exchange for a few crumbs of id satisfaction. I do believe, however, based upon my own insight and the ability that that insight has given me to observe the actions of scores of fellow allergy sufferers, that similar mechanisms and similar stressful situations are much more common than I previously suspected.

**Nothing phony about it**

Over the ten year period prior to my last allergy attack, there had been gradual but meaningful changes taking place in my life. I had become more self-assured and mature. My children were nearly grown. I had become more secure financially. I was content with my occupation and professional status. In other words, slowly, I had eliminated much of the stress that was present at the outset of my affliction.

Although my personal life had improved and stabilized, that did not mean an end yet was in sight for my allergies. I had become so used to the anxiety response that I continued the habit even when there was no apparent reason for it. Old habits—especially bad ones—die hard. I do believe, however, that I finally was prepared emotionally to embark upon a program of exploration and discovery that would bring my affliction under control.

**Old habits die hard**

My last attack occurred during a management convention held in Miami, Florida, in April of 1979. When I boarded the plane for Miami, I had a fever of about 101 and I was suffering from every conceivable allergy symptom. Not only was I miserable, but so was everyone around me. My wife tried her best to enjoy the trip, but she didn't have a chance.

One of the speakers at the convention was Dr. Joyce Brothers. Every time she was about to make an important point or to reach a concluding thought, I would have to sneeze, cough, or blow my nose. I'm sure that Dr. Brothers shall never forget that lecture!

When I returned home from Miami, my attack continued unabated. On April 15, I had *had* it. "Enough," I said to myself. The One-Ten-Ten Method was about to be born.

**Enough is enough**

For additional information regarding the status of current scientific knowledge about the relationship between personality traits and allergy, I strongly recommend that you turn to the Publisher's Supplement in the back of this book and read G. Edward Griffin's revealing chapter entitled *A Suspicious Profile.* If you are *not* interested in the scientific research that has been done along these lines, then you may wish to skip over that material and move directly to Chapter Four.

# IV

# THE METHOD IS BORN

*A review of the events and rationale*
*that culminated in the creation of*
*The One-Ten-Ten Method; initial*
*experience with the method;*
*decision to publish.*

On April 15, 1979, I was experiencing one of the worst allergy attacks to date. As I tried to relax on a chaise lounge in our back yard, sneezing, wheezing, and coughing, a wave of frustration and anger began to sweep over me. Why did this have to happen to *me?* Why should *anyone* have to live in this condition?

As I lay there feeling sorry for myself, I began to reflect on my ten-year battle, and a montage of thoughts and images began to appear on my mental screen. Faces of friends and acquaintances popped into view and repeated their lines: *It's all in your mind!* I replayed my performance at Live Oaks and dwelled for a long time on the possibility that these faces might be speaking the truth.

Then my mental channels began to change. I recalled a recent television program I had seen dealing with hypnosis as one means of treating allergies. Then I remembered an incident that had taken place several years previously at one of our management meetings. One of the guest speakers had been a professional

A TV program
on hypnosis

hypnotist who lectured on the importance of having positive images in our subconscious mind as a prerequisite for success in business. He put on a rather convincing demonstration, and those of us who were in attendance became firm believers.

**The power of suggestion**     At one point in the demonstration, the hypnotist kept repeating: "When you go to bed this evening, you will close your eyes and sleep more soundly than you ever have slept before in your life. When you awake, you will feel strong and refreshed, vital and alert."

It worked! I was feeling vital and alert and literally "hell on wheels" for several days, and I had never slept better in my life.

Recalling these events, my mind flashed across all the things I had ever heard about hypnosis, autosuggestion, or mind-control, and by this time my mental juices were really flowing. Why couldn't they control *allergies* with the power of autosuggestion? It seemed odd to me that, at least to my knowledge, no one had tried this approach.

I knew that it is possible for some people to have needles poked into their skin without feeling pain. How do they do it? Mind Control.

How do people lose weight or quit smoking? Mind Control.

**Mind Control**     Why do humans tend to forget unpleasant experiences? Mind Control.

Realizing that the mind can be a powerful healing instrument, I decided to try to tap my own mind to see what it could do about controlling my allergies. Since I was already in a relaxed state as a result of a belly full of antihistamines, I did not begin with the relaxing exercises that were developed later. (More about that in the next chapter.)

**Borrowing proven phrases**     I recalled the hypnotist's phrases used to implant the suggestion for sleep and vitality, so I used that as a model. Working with the numbers one through ten, I began counting. I substituted the words *I* and *my* in place of *you* and *your,* and, instead of counting backwards from ten to one with the number one being the signal for termination of mental concentration, I simply counted forward from one to ten and repeated the number ten.

Much to my delight, I felt immediate relief after completing the exercise and decided to repeat it four times that same day. After each occasion, I felt physically better.

At the very beginning of this new regimen, I still experienced an occasional sneeze, but, instead of taking handfuls of antihistamines, which had been my usual custom, I was able to manage with only three antihistamines during the first two weeks. That was only one every four days.

As the weeks progressed and I tinkered with the exact wording of the method itself to make it more effective, my condition continued to improve. There no longer was any doubt about it, The One-Ten-Ten Method really worked. After all those years and all that agony, I could hardly believe that the solution had been so simple.

During the month of October, 1979, I called my allergist to verify my peak allergy seasons. He confirmed that they were, as I well knew from experience, spring and fall. It was October. I had just passed through one of my peak seasons. I had quit taking drugs and injections during a peak season. Not only did I pass through this season without an allergy *attack,* I hadn't even experienced any *symptoms.* I had felt no need for an injection or a pill. In fact, I felt then—as now—"Great!"

It was then that I realized the magnitude of what I had stumbled across, and I determined to put the whole thing in writing so that others could have a chance to share in the benefits of my discovery.

Goodby symptoms

# V

# THE ONE-TEN-TEN METHOD

*Step-by-step instructions on how to prepare oneself for successfully applying the method; selecting the right location; how to relax; how to breathe; specific phrases to be committed to memory. This is the core of the self-imaging program.*

We finally are ready to get down to business. The following pages will outline in very specific detail how to apply The One-Ten-Ten Method. It is important that you not be distracted while you read this section. Small details can make a big difference, and you should give this your total, undivided attention. Keep in mind that the method is a technique for development of the subconscious mind. Through it, you will be creating new brain pathways and new mental habits which will enable your subconscious mind to control and relieve the symptoms associated with your allergy. The specific objective of this exercise is to re-program the hypo-thalamus region of your brain to detour your allergy symptoms to another focal point where you will not experience the same reaction. Total concentration is absolutely necessary for you to succeed.

With this in mind, it is easy to see why preparation for the method is just as important as the method itself. You will have to be in the proper state of mind and in the

**Total concentration**

proper environment. There are, undoubtedly, many different techniques that can be used, but I have found the following to be the most effective.

**Isolation**     Isolation is very important, particularly at first or with those who are not used to blocking out mental distractions around them. Isolation, therefore, is helpful as an aid to deep concentration. Generally speaking, any quiet location will suffice. A quiet room where you will not be disturbed for approximately fifteen minutes would be the ideal location for this exercise.

**Positive state of mind**     Next, you must be in a positive state of mind. That means that you must get rid of any negative thoughts or emotions. You must not only *want* the exercise to work for you, you must *expect* it to work for you. If you really believe that you will experience relief, then you already have won most of the battle and are ready to begin.

**Relaxation**     Total relaxation is the third requirement. You must make yourself comfortable and *relax!* This is absolutely essential in order to achieve and maintain concentration. I have found the following steps to be effective and recommend them highly.

**Position is not important**

1.  Make yourself comfortable. You can either sit in a chair with a high back to support your head or you can lie down, according to your preference. The position makes no difference. Just relax and make yourself comfortable.

**Spreading your relaxation**

2.  Close your eyes and concentrate on relaxing your body. Start with your toes on your left foot and, just as soon as you are aware that they are relaxed, move your concentration to your foot; after your foot is relaxed, move to your calf, your thigh, and so on, continuing counter-clockwise, until your entire body is relaxed. Do not

proceed until your entire body is genuinely relaxed.

3.  Introduce soothing images into your mind.    **Soothing images**
    Limit these to scenes associated with soft
    pastel colors, such as light green or light
    blue. Visualize trees, calm water, puffy
    white clouds, or pastural scenes.

4.  Regulate your breathing to simulate that of    **Breathe slowly**
    a sleeping person: slow and regular. If you
    are experiencing breathing difficulties be-
    cause of your allergies, or if you have
    sensitivity in your nasal passages, and
    these are interfering with your ability to
    relax and concentrate, then changing your
    breathing pattern will help. Simply:

**INHALE THROUGH YOUR MOUTH
EXHALE THROUGH YOUR NOSE**

This will relieve your nasal sensitivities.
The substance that was making your nose
more sensitive no longer will be inhaled
through the nose and cannot have the same
effect because of the alternative breathing
pattern.

We are ready now for the phrases themselves—and a word of caution. In order for The One-Ten-Ten Method to have full effectiveness, the following instructions must be followed *exactly as given*. Every word is there for a reason. It is suggested, therefore, that you commit the method to memory.

All words and numbers are to be repeated out loud or silently, depending on your preference.

1. MY MIND IS IN COMMAND OF MY
   BODY. MY MIND IS CONTROLLING ALL
   OF MY BODILY FUNCTIONS.
   Relax and concentrate until you feel as though
   your entire body is being controlled by your
   mind's power. Then continue to number two.

2. I DO NOT HAVE ALLERGIES. I'VE NEVER
   HAD ALLERGIES.
   Relax and concentrate for several moments.
   Then continue to number three.

3. ALL SENSITIVITY IN MY NOSE AND
   EYES WILL MOVE TO MY SCALP.
   Relax and concentrate. Move all of your mental energy to your nose and eyes. As soon as
   you have total concentration in this area, concentrate on removing that sensitivity from your
   nose and eyes, up your forehead, and to your
   scalp. Mentally visualize this movement. As
   soon as you feel the movement or a tingling
   sensation in your scalp go to number four.

4. MY MIND IS IN COMMAND OF MY
   BODY.
   Pause and concentrate
   I AM FEELING BETTER THAN I HAVE
   EVER FELT BEFORE IN MY LIFE.
   Pause and concentrate
   I DO NOT HAVE ALLERGIES. I'VE NEVER
   HAD ALLERGIES.
   Relax and concentrate for several moments.
   Then continue to number five.

5. I DO NOT HAVE ALLERGIES. I'VE NEVER HAD ALLERGIES. I WILL NEVER SNEEZE AGAIN.

    Relax and concentrate for several moments. Then go to number six.

6. ALL SENSITIVITY IN MY NOSE AND EYES WILL MOVE TO MY SCALP.

    Relax and concentrate. Move all of your mental energy to your nose and eyes. As soon as you have total concentration in this area, concentrate on moving the sensitivity from your nose and eyes, up your forehead, and to your scalp. Mentally visualize this movement. As soon as you feel the movement or a tingling sensation in your scalp, go to number seven.

7. MY MIND IS IN COMMAND OF MY BODY.

    Pause and concentrate.

    I AM FEELING BETTER THAN I HAVE EVER FELT BEFORE IN MY LIFE.

    Pause and concentrate.

    I WILL NEVER SNEEZE AGAIN.

    Pause and concentrate.

    MY MIND IS IN COMMAND OF MY BODY.

    Relax and concentrate for several moments. Then go to number eight.

8. I DO NOT HAVE ALLERGIES. I'VE NEVER HAD ALLERGIES. ALL SENSITIVITY IN MY NOSE AND EYES WILL MOVE TO MY SCALP.

    Relax and once again concentrate all of your mental energy to your nose and eyes, and again mentally visualize the movement of sensitivity to your scalp. After you feel the movement or tingling sensation in your scalp, go to number nine.

9. MY MIND IS IN TOTAL COMMAND OF MY BODY. WHEN I SAY THE WORD *TEN*, ALL OF MY MENTAL ENERGY WILL BE CONCENTRATED IN MY NOSE AND EYES. ALL SENSITIVITY IN MY NOSE AND EYES WILL MOVE TO MY SCALP. AFTER I REPEAT THE WORD *TEN*, I WILL OPEN MY EYES AND FEEL BETTER THAN I HAVE EVER FELT BEFORE IN MY LIFE.

Relax and concentrate for several moments. Then go to number ten.

10. All of your mental energy now is concentrated in your nose and eyes. Mentally visualize the sensitivity as it moves from your nose and eyes to your scalp. When you feel the movement or a tingling in your scalp, hold your concentration there for several moments. Now repeat the word

### TEN!

After opening your eyes, you should feel relaxed and refreshed, better than you have ever felt before in your life.

**The importance of ten**     At this point you may be wondering about certain features of The One-Ten-Ten Method. Some people, for example, ask "Why did he use the numbers 1-10-10?", or "Why did he use words such as *I* or *my* instead of *you* or *your*?" or "Why did he select the scalp as a focal point?"

The number series *1-10-10* was used for several reasons. First of all, we mentally associate many things with the numbers one through ten. For example: the ten count in boxing, counting to ten when angry, counting to ten in the game of hide and seek. The first number series learned as a child is one through ten. In mathematics, the multiple of ten is the basic unit for all higher numbers. The number ten, therefore, has a great many subconscious reinforcements. We can easily identify with these numbers, which is why they have been selected as points of reference.

The specific words used in The One-Ten-Ten Method have been selected because they are clear and can be committed to memory in a relatively short period of time. The words *you* and *your* were rejected because I believe that, when someone says "you're going to do this," or "you will do that," human nature often will cause us to resist the command and want to do just the opposite. This problem is avoided when we think *I* will do so and so because *I* want to do it.

**Choosing the right words**

The scalp was selected as the sensitivity transfer point because of two reasons. First, it is located relatively close to the region of the nose and eyes, where most of the symptoms of hay fever are concentrated, and it is relatively easy to mentally move these symptoms just the short distance up the forehead and to the scalp. The other reason is that the scalp is a part of the body where it would be impossible for the same kind of allergy reaction to occur. For most people, therefore, the scalp is an ideal repository of symptom concentration. For those with allergies other than hay fever or bronchial asthma, I suggest that you apply the following techniques to your specific condition.

**The role of the scalp**

Where the method makes reference to the nose and eyes, simply substitute the word or phrase that best describes the nature or location of your allergy.

For example, refer to number eight of the method. Assuming your allergy takes the form of a rash or hives, after repeating "I do not have allergies. I've never had allergies," then say "All sensitivity from my *rash* will move to my scalp *and exit through my hair follicles.*"

**The value of color**     One further alternative may be of value to you. If you find that you have trouble moving your sensitivity, you may be more successful if you assign a *color* to it. In other words, in your mind's eye, identify the color blue, yellow, or green—the choice is entirely up to you—to your sensitivity and work with that. This may help your concentration by giving you something definite upon which to focus your thoughts. This works quite well for many people.

Once you have a clear understanding of the One-Ten-Ten Method and have committed its content to memory, relax, close your eyes, concentrate, and follow the required sequence.

You may now begin.

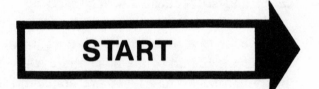

## 1.

My mind is in command of my body.

My mind is controlling all of my bodily functions.

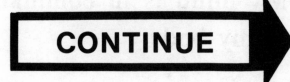

## 2.

I do not have allergies.

I've never had allergies.

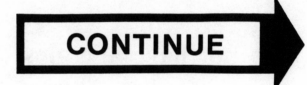

# 3.

# All sensitivity in my nose and eyes will move to my scalp.

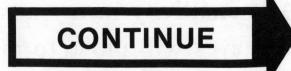

**4.**

My mind is in command of my body.

I am feeling better than I have ever felt before in my life.

I do not have allergies.

I've never had allergies.

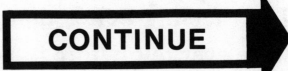

5.

I do not have allergies.

I've never had allergies.

I will never sneeze again.

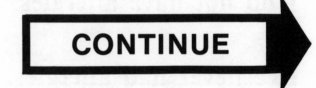

6.

All sensitivity in my nose
and eyes will move to my
scalp.

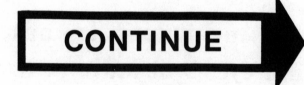

7.

My mind is in command
of my body.

I am feeling better than I
have ever felt before in my
life.

I will never sneeze again.

My mind is in command
of my body.

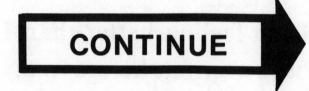

## 8.

I do not have allergies.

I've never had allergies.

All sensitivity in my nose and eyes will move to my scalp.

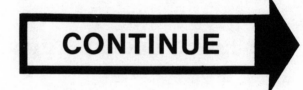

## 9.

My mind is in total command of my body.

When I say the word *ten*, all of my mental energy will be concentrated in my nose and eyes.

All sensitivity in my nose and eyes will move to my scalp.

After I repeat the word *ten*, I will open my eyes and feel better than I have ever felt before in my life.

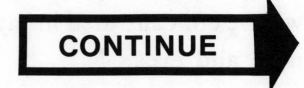

# 10.

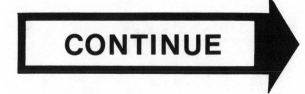

# TEN.

The entire exercise should take approximately ten to fifteen minutes. It should be applied in accordance with the following schedule.

WEEKS ONE AND TWO: Repeat the method three times a day: once in the morning, once in the afternoon, and, if the afternoon sequence is not possible because of unavailability of isolation, then once early in the evening and once before going to bed.

WEEKS THREE AND FOUR: Repeat the method twice a day, once in the morning and once in the evening.

MONTHS TWO AND THREE: Repeat the method once a day. If you should feel yourself losing control, then go back to twice a day.

MONTHS FOUR AND FIVE: Repeat the method every other day. If you should feel yourself losing control, then go back to once a day.

MONTH SIX: From this point on, use as needed.

As I have stated previously, the high percentage of success of The One-Ten-Ten Method has been both astounding and gratifying. It is self-evident, however, that it is not a cure-all. It is intended as an alternative or supplement to conventional treatment, depending on circumstances. Undoubtedly, there are people who, for one reason or another, will not find relief with this program. For example, an infant or a very young child will not have the power of concentration. (A special audio cassette recording has been developed as an aid to those who may have difficulty reading or concentrating. Please see the back of this book for details.) Persons with severe emotional problems, likewise, may find it impossible to totally relax or to concentrate. Common sense dictates that, in these cases, specialists in childhood allergies or psychological counselors should be sought.

For a significant segment of the allergy population, however, The One-Ten-Ten Method will be extremely helpful. If you are among this number, you will discover that, even if there is an occasional sneeze or cough, you will be able to control your symptoms and lead a normal life once again.

I feel extremely fortunate that, by a happy combination of events and personal experiences, I had been exposed to the bits and dabs of information that eventually fell into place as pieces of the allergy puzzle. It was mostly sheer luck on my part; certainly not a result of any great talent or scientific genius in the field of allergy research. Now that The One-Ten-Ten Method is developed, however, I am delighted at the prospects of sharing my good fortune with the untold numbers of allergy sufferers throughout the world. And so, especially to you who have diligently read these pages, I wish you...

Good luck and good health!

# VI

# THE GOOD NEWS SPREADS

*Early experiments by others with
The One-Ten-Ten Method;
first-person testimonials from
allergy sufferers who found relief;
unexpected demand for copies of the
method; interest from the press.*

While I was putting together my notes for publication of The One-Ten-Ten Method, I still had reservations about its overall utility. I knew that it worked for *me*, and it seemed logical that it should work for others, but I really didn't know for certain. In order to resolve this question, I distributed copies of my preliminary draft of the manuscript to people who were suffering from hay fever, asthma, and related allergies. Some of these people apparently were sufficiently comfortable with their condition that they lacked the motivation to give my program a try. On the other hand, the results from the people who did try the method were absolutely astounding. Without a single exception, those who tried it and believed it would help them, all experienced positive results. With their consent, I would like to share their victories with you at this time.

The first letter I want to enter into the record is one of the most recent ones received. In fact, it was delivered

**The method is tried by others**

Len Mazzuca

only a few days before the manuscript was scheduled for the typesetter. It is especially interesting because of the almost instantaneous success of the method. It came from Mr. Len Mazzuca of Canoga Park, California, and reads as follows:

TO WHOM IT MAY CONCERN:

I have had allergies all of my life. The doctors told me that I would outgrow it. I know now that I will not outgrow this, so I have relied on [antihistamine] to help me through the bad times. Lately, it seems that even this is not helping.

With the thought of something new to try, I was most interested when John Laccinole gave me the The One-Ten-Ten Method and I was happy to give it my best. I have been involved in self-hypnosis before as an aid in selling techniques, and the method sounded interesting.

As I was relaxing during my first experiment with The One-Ten-Ten Method, I could feel the process working on the concentrated area right away. The tingling was definitely there, and I could actually feel the sensitivity moving to my scalp. The next feeling was that of my nasal passages opening up, as if I had taken a couple of [antihistamines]. There are

Just thinking about it brings relief

times now when I feel an attack coming on, and just thinking about the method has proved a relief to me. Yet, I have only had access to the method for four days and have not given it a real chance.

My ten-year old daughter sat down last night and asked if she, too, could try it, because she has the same allergies. After we were through, she said she could feel a difference and that she had some relief. Both of us agreed we did feel more comfortable and relaxed afterwards, which I feel has a lot to do with the overall symptoms.

I can't wait to tell my brother of this, as he, too, has the same problems....

I am most appreciative of John Laccinole who discussed The One-Ten-Ten Method with me and encouraged me to try it. I intend to continue because I can see the potential and the help for an old problem that will soon be gone.

One of the most gratifying cases involved an eleven-year old boy with near crippling hay fever. His name is Wally Jukes, and he lives in Canoga Park, California. The following series of letters tell the story. On March 11, 1980, Rhonda Jukes, Wally's mother, wrote to me and said:

**Wally Jukes**

> We introduced our eleven-year old son to The One-Ten-Ten Method as an alternative treatment for allergies. Since that time, we have experienced miraculous results. As an active child, Wally would come in from play or school completely out of breath, almost unable to breathe. Wally had been under the doctor's care for the last eight years and had received the usual treatment and prescriptions. Now, with The One-Ten-Ten plan he no longer requires either doctors or prescriptions which is a miracle. This change is so dramatic he can go play Little League baseball without medication or the usual pocket full of tissues at the height of his allergy season!
>
> Since Wally has just turned eleven, I might add, he does not always practice One-Ten-Ten the prescribed three times per day. Usually it takes a sneeze or two to get him to follow the procedure, but it works every time. Once we thoroughly explained to him that he was in

**No more doctors or prescriptions**

control and didn't need pills, he became excited about it. We spent some time working with him so he'd fully understand the program, which we believe was very important. Now, when there is lots of pollen in the air, Wally's response is quick (using One-Ten-Ten) and the results are always the same, no problems!

One month later, on April 9, 1980, Mrs. Jukes wrote to me again, granting permission to use her statements regarding her son's progress, and she added:

**Still breathes the same air**

Wally is doing better than ever at present. As a matter of fact, we regard his allergies as a thing of the past. Wally's pediatrician had diagnosed him as having hay fever and basically being allergic to almost everything in the air. Needless to say, he is still breathing the same air, but now he has his body under control through The One-Ten-Ten Method.

Two months later, in a letter dated June 27, 1980, Mrs. Jukes commented further:

Wally is doing extremely well with The One-Ten-Ten Method. He still has not seen a doctor or taken any medication (prescription or otherwise) since he started using the method. He has not had any allergy attacks, either. At this point, I would like to thank John Laccinole for making us "aware" of this method, but I want to thank Wally for executing the method and achieving his goals! The method does nothing unless what is learned is lived....I asked Wally to comment on his experience with and thoughts on The One-Ten-Ten Method, so please find enclosed his letter which I have left unedited.

Wally's letter, as written in his own handwriting, was short and to the point:

Dear Sir,

 When I started your program I was ten. **Success at age ten**
Now I am eleven and I do this program twice a day. I feel really good when I do The One-Ten-Ten Method. I can breathe now, except when I get nervous. Then I start sneezing, but I have been working on it. If a person had allergy, I would recommend it to that person, because it has worked for me. Whenever I do The One-Ten-Ten Method, I feel better and better each time I do it. I can change my focal point to anywhere. When I began, I could hardly get my scalp to feel it. Now I hardly have any allergy. It worked for me because I got familiar with it and did it right.

     Your friend, Wally Jukes

I mentioned previously that my own mother suffered from allergies. I since have learned that this is extremely common. It was uncanny how so many of those first users of The One-Ten-Ten Method were adults who, immediately after obtaining positive results for themselves, introduced the method to their own children.

 Maria de la Luz Monarrez was typical in this regard. She **Maria de la Luz** wrote a long letter to me on April 10, 1980, recounting **Monarrez** her life-long battle against allergies. The highlights of that letter are as follows:

Dear Mr. Laccinole,

 I am thirty-five years old, married, and have three daughters, ages fourteen, twelve, and ten. I was born with allergies. The bronchial asthma did not come about until I was about ten or so.

My school years were spent blowing my nose and sneezing. I had constant eye and throat infections, swollen glands, and very itchy ears.... It was hard for my dad to accept the fact that he had a "sick" daughter. In those days, being healthy was more than normal, it was an honor. I often was made to feel as a **Treated as a freak** freak....

I still remember my first asthmatic attack. My family had gone to the drive-in in the family station wagon...to see "Phantom of the Opera," one of my favorites. Not long after we arrived, my chest started hurting every time I coughed. I could feel the tightness in the chest increasing and it was getting harder for me to breathe. I tried to tell my mom, but nothing came out. She saw the fear in my eyes and told my dad. He couldn't be bothered. He felt I was just getting a chest cold. I spent the rest of the evening scared and in pain. We didn't leave until the movie ended.

To make a long story short, I was finally taken to emergency hours later. My dad drove us there but stayed in the car. My mom and I went in. It was a few more hours before I was seen. (Since I was not confirmed as an asthmatic, I was considered an "emotional asthmatic")....

I have spent my life with a handkerchief in my hand and a purse full of pills and sprays along with an inhaler for asthma. My medicine cabinet looks like a pharmacy. My attempts at gardening, riding a bike, or just enjoying the sun have proven futile. (I also have allergy to the sun.)...

**Four shots every week** I've been tested five times in the last seven years. Have had four injections a week, every week. Went down to three shots a week for a while. Was retested on April 9, 1980. Due to the results, *new allergies!* I'm now back to four shots every week....

Since I first talked to you, I've been able to prevent three asthma attacks, one of them while driving on the freeway. Your technique has also enabled me to get over stress by helping me to relax.... Your method came to my aid yesterday when I was being retested for allergies. Ordinarily, my nose is running terribly during the testing. While waiting results on my arms. I relaxed and kept telling myself I had no allergies. My test results were bad, but my nose only became stuffed for a few minutes. I did not have to take an antihistamine immediately following the testing. The hour drive home was only mildly uncomfortable compared to prior testing....

A special thanks to my friend Bonnie who cared enough to introduce me to you and to your method.

That letter obviously was written only a short time after Mrs. Monarrez had started the program. Two and a half months later, on June 23, 1980, she wrote with considerably more enthusiasm:

Two weeks ago, my sister and I went to help our parents clean their house. They're both disabled and there was much to do. I usually wheeze a lot while dusting. I felt the wheezing start, took time out to do my "exercise" (The One-Ten-Ten Method) and felt fine the rest of the day.

**Overcoming house dust**

Last week, my youngest daughter, Natalie, wanted me to go bike riding with her. Since she and I were the only two at home, I said OK. Our tract is on a hill, and the streets are not flat. My legs hurt a lot, but my breathing was fine. I didn't even sneeze!

My husband, Rudy, is a firefighter for Los Angeles County and is very active in sports. At the moment, he is managing a softball team and running competition in firemens' musters. His activities sure get us around.

**The Hose Cart Competition**

On May 24th, we were in Ukiah for a muster. One of the events was "Womens' Hose Cart Competition." I was asked to compete. I said no. Not having run since school days, I was more afraid of what could happen. My husband and friends convinced me to give it a trial run. I was "nozzle person." I was to help push a hose cart (while running as fast as I could) one-hundred feet, then grab the nozzle and attach it to the hose coupling being held by my partner. At this point, I straighten the hose, then get on top of my partner who is already flat on her stomach holding the hose nozzle. Our combined weight is to keep the pressure of the water that is coming through the hose from going in any other direction but where it is aimed. When the water comes, I am to help direct the nozzle toward the cone that we are trying to knock down. It is a timed event and a lot of fun to watch.

**A real victory**

After the practice run, I found myself sitting in the street (where we ran) exhausted and wheezing. I did my five-minute "exercise," then felt fine. Needless to say, I went ahead and did the actual run. Our team came in seventh place out of nineteen womens' teams. We did not win, but I felt quite a winner.

At this point, Mrs. Monarrez included a report on her oldest daughter, Roselyn, age fourteen, who also had been introduced to The One-Ten-Ten Method. The report reads as follows:

> She has had bronchial asthma and allergies since birth. Has been given allergy tests and gets four shots every four to six weeks.... Due to allergies, she has been unable to participate in many outdoor activities.... She has experimented with many different make-ups, as some cause her face to develop a rash. She also has food allergies which greatly upset her stomach. When exam day came around at school, she always had bad hay fever symptoms and would need medication from the school nurse. She later started doing the "exercise" just before exam time and found that she felt fine. Stress played a big role.
>
> This summer, my daughters have taken up jogging. Roselyn is doing her best at building up her running time. She was able to run one-and-a-half blocks last week without any problems and hopes to increase that this week.
>
> Her health has improved with the "exercise." She went on a group trip to Magic Mountain last week and did not need any medication.
>
> Her outlook has greatly improved since she started the exercise. She now knows what to do if she starts to have allergy problems and, with time, should be able to live a very normal life....
>
> I had learned to accept my way of life and felt that my allergies rendered me helpless many times because that's the way life was. Now, thanks to Mr. Laccinole and his exercise, I also have much to look forward to.

**Roselyn Monarrez**

**Allergy and school exams**

**A normal life at last**

You can imagine my delight at receiving these letters and reports. I now knew that I was not unique and that The One-Ten-Ten Method was of value, not just to me,

**Good news travels fast**

but to almost anyone who would really give it a try.

They say that bad news travels fast. That may well be true, but I'm here to tell you that *good* news spreads fast, too. As each person succeeded with the program, the word would go out through family and friends in ever-widening circles until it was moving like wildfire. My phone began to ring constantly, and the daily mail brought scores of requests—mostly from people I didn't know—for copies of instructions to the method. Photocopies of my preliminary notes proliferated like black market video copies of first-run movies. News reporters, TV producers, and feature story writers called for interviews.

I was not prepared for this crush and certainly was not interested in getting into a major medical research program involving the collection and evaluation of thousands of case histories. I just wanted to tell as many people as I could exactly how the method works so they could try it themselves. I decided to stop sending out photocopies and, of sheer necessity, even to stop answering the mail so as to devote full energy to the single purpose of getting the whole story into print.

This publication is the product of that effort.

# PUBLISHER'S SUPPLEMENT

Additional research and comments
by G. Edward Griffin.

# A DYNAMITE THEORY

by G. Edward Griffin    ©1980

*Motivation for becoming involved in research; survey of current theories about allergy; case histories suggesting the importance of psychological factors; evidence that allergy is both physiological and psychological; review of the autonomic, sympathetic, and parasympathetic nervous systems; role of the hypothalamus and pituitary gland; experimental studies supportive of the neurological theory of allergy; the use and danger of deep-trance hypnosis; summary and conclusions.*

I'll never forget the day John Laccinole first walked into my office. As a small publishing house we are used to receiving manuscripts that already have been turned down by major publishers. In many cases, it is not difficult to see why they were rejected. We get everything from autobiographical poetry written by taxi cab drivers to revelations from little people in outer space. Laccinole fit in just fine. He dropped a thin sheaf of papers on my desk bearing the unlikely title of *The One-Ten-Ten Method.*

Meeting the author

"I know you're busy," he said, "and I'm kind of in a hurry myself, so I won't waste your time trying to explain it. Just read it. It's dynamite!"

With that, he shook my hand and started to leave. He had been in my office less than three minutes.

"What's it about?" I asked as he moved toward the door.

"Just read it," was the reply. "It's dynamite!" And he was gone.

A week later, Laccinole and I confronted each other for about two hours straight. I had, indeed, read the manuscript, and I was convinced that the author had slipped a cog, but I was intrigued by the possibility that he might really have something. I was determined to find out.

I knew very little about allergies at that time, except that some people have them and some don't. Fortunately, I was in the second catagory. The thought, however, that allergies could be controlled simply by repeating ten simple phrases seemed like nonsense. Yet, Laccinole, himself, was living, walking proof that such an approach worked, at least for *him*. Why not others? Then I learned that others *had* been helped. I read their letters. I met them in person.

**Living proof that it worked**

I called an allergist who also happens to be a close personal friend and asked him what he thought. Much to my surprise, he didn't reject the concept. In fact, he was very open-minded and expressed interest in learning more.

"John, we've decided to publish your book."

"I knew you would," he said matter-of-factly. "It's dynamite, isn't it?"

"But," I replied, "no one will believe that there is a scientific base to your theory. They'll think that it is just a bunch of jibberish coming from someone who has no real knowledge in the field. What this book needs is some solid research of the medical literature to show that The One-Ten-Ten Method *is* scientifically sound.

We want you to do that and put it into the front part of the book."

"Hey, I don't have the *time* for the additional research, but if you want to dig into it yourself and add a publisher's supplement, that's OK with me."

The idea intrigued me. The primary appeal was that it would give me a chance to satisfy my own curiosity on the subject. The one thing I did not want to do was lend my name to something that wasn't scientifically sound. In such matters, there's no substitute for first-hand knowledge based on one's own research. So, with the able help of my wife, Pat, who was good enough to spend the better part of a day at the UCLA Biomedical Library selecting reference books and ordering a computer search of the medical periodicals, I eagerly accepted the challenge and began to dig into the literature. What follows is the result of that survey.

**The lure of a research project**

I presume that most of you who are reading these pages either are allergy sufferers or have a loved one who is. Otherwise, you probably wouldn't have been motivated to acquire this book in the first place. I'm not going to waste your time, therefore, telling you things you already know, such as how widespread allergies are, what the symptoms are, or what traditional treatments are available. Instead, I'm going to jump right into the middle of the subject and deal with the central mystery of why allergies occur. Unless, we can answer that question, it is unlikely that anyone ever will figure out how to *cure* allergies, unless by the most fantastic luck from empirical trial and error.

First of all, let us define terms. It is generally understood that the word *allergy* covers a wide range of symptoms, many of them simulating other diseases. Allergic reactions can affect almost any organ or tissue of the body. Depending on their specific symptom and target organ, they are known as asthma (restricted breathing), hay fever (sneezing and running eyes), allergic rhinitis (running nose), urticaria (hives), eczema

**A definition of terms**

(swollen patches on the skin) gastro-intestinal allergy (colitis and diarrhea), to name just a few. Many allergists also would include migraine headaches among the allergy diseases.[1]

The number of theories about the nature of allergy is approximately equal to the number of writers on the subject. They represent a wide range of viewpoints from a purely physiological (chemical/mechanical) view on the one hand to a classical Freudian (psycho/sexual) view on the other. At the present time, however, the most prevalent professional opinion falls somewhere between the two extremes.

It is important to realize that the entire field of allergy as a science is still relatively new. It is not surprising, therefore, that there should be a great deal of divergence of opinion and that, occasionally, one is confronted by an apparent impasse of conflicting data.

**Chemical/mechanical reactions**     Much has been written about the chemical/mechanical aspect of allergy. Our present understanding is that, for some unknown reason, an individual may become over sensitive to a common substance or environmental condition. Without trying to go into all the technical aspects of the mechanism, suffice it to say that the body's immune/defense system goes haywire. It tries to defend itself against this "allergen" by producing antibodies and by trying to overcome the offending substance or condition through swelling tissue, coughing, sneezing, running nose, or diarrhea.

A lot of chemistry takes place involving natural histamine and cortisone, protein conversion, and that sort of thing. The end result, however, is that our immune system, which is our friend under normal conditions, becomes our enemy.

Why this should happen remains almost as much a mystery today as when the condition was first described by Hippocrates in the year 400 B.C. There is no logic to the fact that so many people should manifest a condition that, under primitive conditions, would seem to act against survival. If this condition did exist in prehistoric man, why didn't it disappear through the process of natural selection? And why are there no observable allergies among the lower animals?

The primary difference between man and the lower animals, of course, is his intellect. Is it possible that this is a clue to the mechanism of allergy? Could man's *brain,* with its capacity for abstraction, imagination, and rationalization be at the core of his allergy problems? Let us consider the following cases taken from the medical literature.

**The brain is suspect**

Dr. Warren T. Vaughan, internationally recognized authority on allergy, reports five interesting cases.[2] A student is allergic to eggs and tomatoes, so he avoids them and all is well. But, when he studies for exams, he gets hives even though he does not eat eggs or tomatoes.

**A survey of cases**

A banker also gets hives from tomatoes, but during the bank "holiday" of the great depression, he, likewise, is covered with hives in the absence of tomatoes.

An asthmatic woman is in an auto accident. Afterward, whenever she is riding and her husband must hit the brakes, she begins to wheeze.

A man has three episodes of hives over a one-year period. He is tested and shown to be allergic to house dust. He is treated each time with shots and the symptoms go away. Later, the allergist learns that each incident coincided with a traumatic encounter in the man's marriage, not with an increase in house dust.

An allergy clinic gives pollen desensitizing shots to many patients each day. The current pollen count is posted on the bulletin board for all to see. One day, when the pollen count is exceptionally low, the staff posts a high count just to see what effect it might have. After reading the false report, several of the patients experienced marked increase in their hay fever symptoms.

Does this prove that it's all in one's head? Certainly not. First of all, not all allergy sufferers respond in this

**It is not all in our heads**

fashion. Secondly, in every case, there either were or could have been allergies responsible for the reactions in addition to the psychological factors. Even those who did not eat their eggs or tomatoes could, in fact, have developed temporary allergic reactions to other substances that normally they could tolerate. It does support the hypothesis, however, that allergic reactions are not solely chemical or physiological in nature. Psychological factors clearly are present and must not be ignored.

Let us move cautiously now to the next step. Is it *possible* that the physical machinery of allergy can be put into motion by psychological factors? Notice that we are not asking if *only* psychological factors are at work, we are asking if the chemical/mechanical reactions, which most assuredly do exist, could, somehow, be triggered by mental factors. There is, in fact, much evidence to support this assumption.

**House dust vs. home environment**

As long ago as 1958, it was reported in a study of severely asthmatic children that, when the children were hospitalized and removed from their home environment, they no longer reacted to their own house dust which was brought in for the test. But, when they returned to their families, their allergic reactions also returned.[3]

**Watermelon and a conditioned reflex**

A woman became highly allergic to watermelon. She could be relatively close to the offending fruit without reaction *if she could not see it.* But let her just get a glimpse of the watermelon across the room and she would have an immediate, violent reaction.[4] The interesting thing about this case is that there is little question of allergens at work. The reaction is triggered by visual stimulus and obviously *originates* in her nervous system. It represents a classical example of conditioned reflex.

**The importance of the nervous system**

The nervous system should not be dismissed lightly when attempting to construct a theoretical model of the allergy mechanism. For example, a tourniquet was placed around the arm of a man with cold hives (blotches produced in reaction to temperatures normally not considered to be severe). Then his hand was dipped into cold water. Immediately the blotches appeared, not just up to the elastic band, but all over his body. Obviously, no chemical substance could have been produced at the site of the cold and then quickly circulated through the blood stream to remote parts of the body; further evidence that the nervous system is intimately involved in allergy reactions.[5]

Let's take a closer look. A rose may be a rose may be a rose, but the nervous system is not all alike. The *central nervous system* is the part that controls our conscious actions and sensations, such as sight, sound, smell, touch, and movement of our limbs. The *autonomic nervous system* is the part that controls our unconscious bodily functions, such as heart beat, dilation of the pupils in the eyes, secretion of saliva, and so on. As you already may have guessed, all of the coughing, sneezing, wheezing, puffing, and blotching that occurs in an allergic reaction is under control of the autonomic nervous system. So let's really zero in on that.

**The central nervous system**

**The autonomic nervous system**

Dr. Warren Vaughan, explains it this way:

Our present interest in the autonomic nervous system is that it controls the activity of smooth muscles, those muscles which become too active during the allergic reaction. This control is maintained by two divisions or sets of these nerves which act antagonistically toward each other—one might say in opposite directions. One set, the *sympathetic,* causes relaxation of certain muscles, while the other, the *parasympathetic,* causes their contraction. The actual state of tonicity of the muscle depends upon relative preponderance of action of the two nerves. The allergic shock tissues are controlled by these two opposed groups of

**The sympathetic and parasympathetic systems**

nerves. Under normal conditions, in a state of inactivity, the two sets are equally active and the muscle is at rest, neither highly contracted or abnormally relaxed. Under conditions of physiological activity, one nerve system or the other becomes dominant.[6]

Don't go away. We are getting close to the core of the problem. What happens when the sympathetic nervous system becomes dominant?

Dr. Vaughan answers:

**The origin of allergic responses**

It is the sympathetic system which in great measure controls our adjustment to our environment. It controls the protective reactions. As long as it has the upper hand we need have no fear of allergic responses. It is when the parasympathetic gets control that we experience difficulty adjusting....Adaptation to environmental problems may fail because of underactivity of the sympathetic system or because of overactivity of the parasympathetic. This latter is what appears to happen in allergy.[7]

Let's see what we have here. The allergy response mechanism may be caused by over-stimulation of the parasympathetic nervous system. But just where is this alleged "system" and how might it be overstimulated?

The "system," of course, is distributed throughout the body, but it all comes together in the brain. No one really knows for certain how it is stimulated, but it is **The pituitary gland** likely that the pituitary gland is at least one of the regulators and, like the guy who wakes up the bugler, it is the hypothalamus segment of the brain that regulates the pituitary.

Dr. Harold Michal-Smith, Associate Professor of Clinical Psychiatry at New York Medical College, tells us:

A possible biochemical explanation for psychological effects in allergy may lie in the effect of psychological stress upon the pituitary adrenocortical axis. Neurological studies have provided sufficient evidence that the site of emotional generation is in the hypothalamus, and that stimuli generated there affect the adjacent pituitary gland, which in turn affects corticosteroid secretion.[8]

**The hypothalamus**

The significance of this to the allergy victim is that, once the pituitary gland has stimulated the parasympathetic nervous system, the allergy trigger mechanism becomes cocked and can be released by the slightest change in environment.

Dr. Vaughan tells us:

When a shock tissue has developed the habit of responding to stimulation by an allergen, the trigger mechanism is set, and nonallergenic stimulation may set it off. A person whose hay fever is due to house dust and whose trigger mechanism is set may sneeze from the irritation of ordinary road dust, from looking at the bright sun, from infection in the sinuses, and even from emotional upsets. The autonomic nervous system is connected directly with the brain and the trigger may be released by nerve impulses as well as by external irritants. Indeed, the person who sneezes when looking at the sun could do so only because of transmission of the stimulus from the eye to the nose by way of the nerves.[9]

**The allergy trigger**

So here we have a working model at last. Emotional stress triggers the hypothalamus. The hypothalamus activates the pituitary. The pituitary stimulates the parasympathetic nervous system causing an imbalance

**A working model**

in the autonomic nervous system. This results in a predisposition of the smooth muscles associated with allergy symptoms to contract at the slightest provocation. This condition expresses itself as an over sensitization to substances or environmental conditions that normally would cause no reaction, and this lowered threshold of tolerance to miniscule irritants is known as **The prime mover** allergy. Thus, we can see the prime mover in the entire **is stress** chain reaction is stress. The pollens and cat hairs, the protein molecules and temperature extremes, even the malfunction in the production of antibodies, these are but accessories to the crime. They become involved in the process, to be sure, but they are merely the lackeys of the big boss who gives the orders: Emotional Stress.

If this theory is correct, we would expect to observe certain phenomena among allergy sufferers. For **Logical expectations** example, we would expect that anything that increased emotional stress would increase allergy symptoms even though the particular allergen to which the patient is sensitive is reduced or eliminated. We would expect, conversely, that anything that reduces emotional stress would reduce allergy symptoms even though the allergen exposure is the same or greater. Finally, we would expect that many allergy victims not only would be sensitive to different kinds of allergens (remember, its the reduced tolerance to irritants, not the irritants themselves), but that they also would experience more than one type of allergy, that asthmatics often could become afflicted with hives, and so forth. All of this, in fact, is exactly what the record shows.

A study released in 1976 reported that, when chronic asthmatic children were asked to concentrate on **The effect of anger** remembered incidents of intense anger or fear, their **or fear** breathing flow rates, which were being measured by scientific instruments, became significantly reduced. Since their exposure to allergens remained unchanged during the experiment, only the stress factor can explain the increase of symptoms.[10]

In another study dealing with patients with urticaria (hives), both psychological testing and electroencephalograms (brain wave readings) were used to determine stress levels. It was found that, in the majority of cases, "first symptoms coincided with frustrating situations and psychic stress-intensified manifestations." Eighty-two per cent of the patients had abnormal brain waves typical of high stress patterns.[11]

**The effect of frustration and stress**

One of the early experiments along this line was conducted in Canada and published in 1952. A group of asthmatic children was given psychological therapy and then measured for symptom severity. The results were astounding. The symptoms had decreased between fifty and one-hundred per cent.[12]

In the case of young children with asthma, it is logical to assume that the primary source of emotional stress is to be found somewhere in the home or family environment. It could be conflict with parent, with rival brothers or sisters, or a host of other interactions, most of which are not consciously perceived by the family members themselves. The following experiment, therefore, was particularly significant. A group of asthmatic children was divided randomly into two. The experimental group received family psychotherapy over a four-month period. The control group had none. Both groups continued to receive standard medical treatments. The group with family psychotherapy showed significant improvement compared to the control group.[13]

**The effect of psychological counseling**

Results have been even more encouraging at the adult level. A group of asthma victims ranging in age from twenty to fifty-five was given autogenic (self-hypnosis) training. They practiced using their mind to alter bodily functions that normally are considered to be automatic. In other words, they become proficient at bridging the gap between the central nervous system (conscious) and the autonomic nervous system (subconscious). At the completion of their training, they were compared with a control group taken at random from the same larger pool

**The effect of self-hypnosis**

from which the experimental group had been drawn. Here are the results. During the summer high-pollen season, from April through November, the control group experienced a decrease of ability to breathe by ten to twenty per cent. The patients receiving autogenic training, however, enjoyed an *increase* in the ability to breathe by twenty-two to twenty-seven per cent! A follow-up study showed that the autogenic group as a whole had missed 663 days from work in the year prior to training, but only 77 days in the year following training. That's an improvement of over eighty-eight per cent.[14]

**Multiple allergies are common**

Is it true that allergy victims often exchange one type of allergy for another or that they may sustain several at the same time? The answer is yes. A study by Dr. Warren Vaughan and Dr. Harvey Black showed that fifty nine per cent of eczema patients also developed respiratory allergies.[15] Dr. Michal-Smith confirms this fact and then adds:

> Actually, in the same individual the shock organ, that is the skin or the lungs, may alternate from time to time. For this type of alternate manifestation, Ratner[16] and his associates originated the term "dermal-respiratory syndrome." It is not uncommon practice to note that, as the skin of an individual with eczema clears, asthma may develop.[17]

**Eczema improved by biofeedback**

This is strong support for the neurological theory of allergy, for there simply is no other theory at present that can explain this phenomenon. But perhaps the most convincing evidence of all comes from yet another study in biofeedback techniques. A group of eczema patients actually was trained to increase or decrease the electrical conductivity of their own skin. Since skin conductance is related to tissue water content, the patients were, in reality, manipulating the water content of the cells in and beneath their skin. This is precisely the mechanism that, when it fails to function properly, results in eczema. It is not surprising, therefore, that those patients who learned to decrease skin conductance (and water content) also showed clinical improvement in their disease. But the hidden bonus was that they also showed a reduction of *anxiety*.[18]

I once saw a stage hypnotist convince a woman that she was allergic to her husband. I personally knew the couple, by the way, so I can vouch for the fact that the incident was not staged. When she was awakened from her trance, she had no conscious recollection of the post-hypnotic suggestion. When she returned to her seat in the audience next to her husband, she suddenly began to sneeze violently. Her eyes puffed up almost immediately and her nose began to flow. The hypnotist asked the husband to come to the stage to get an article belonging to the woman which he purposely had kept as an excuse to separate the couple momentarily. As soon as the man left his seat, his wife's symptoms began to clear up, but when he returned, the poor woman became convulsed in her new allergy once again. With a snap of the hypnotist's fingers, all was returned to normal.

**Allergy induced by hypnotism**

There are several lessons to be learned from this event that are important. First, as far as the woman was concerned, the temporary allergy was *real*. There was absolutely no difference between her symptoms and those of an individual who might be overly sensitive to ragweed or house dust. Second, it was *not* all in her head. Her eyes puffed up, her nose ran, she sneezed, and for all I knew she may even have developed hives which I merely failed to observe. In any event, her symptoms were very physical in nature. Third, she *was* allergic to her husband, or at least to something associated with him. It could have been the odor of his hair tonic, shaving cream, or even natural body oil. Whatever it was, it probably was so insignificant as to be unnoticed by others, certainly not offensive. Yet, it became an irritant that her body simply could not tolerate. Fourth,

**Psychologically induced but physically real**

and perhaps most important of all, is the conclusion that, if a real, physical allergy can be *created* by the mind, it should be able to be *controlled* by the mind. I didn't realize it at the time, but the hypnotist had demonstrated the rationale for the One-Ten-Ten Method.

**Allergies controlled by hypnotherapy**

As one might expect, studies in clinical hypnotherapy have produced some very encouraging statistics. One such experiment on a group of children, ages six to seventeen, each with bronchial asthma, showed an average overall symptom improvement of more than fifty per cent.[19] A similar hypnotherapy experiment on adult asthmatic patients resulted in thirty-three per cent with definite improvement plus another twenty-one per cent that became *completely free* from asthma and required no further drug therapy.[20]

**A word of caution**

As favorable as these results may be, the use of deep-trance hypnotherapy should be approached with extreme caution. If a patient's allergy is the result of a profound, repressed psychological conflict, then using hypnosis to remove the allergy in effect will remove the outlet for the suppressed conflict. The result could be a sudden exchange of the allergy mechanism for another far more dangerous or socially unacceptable behavior pattern. It is important to note at this point that, while The One-Ten-Ten Method *is* a form of autosuggestion, it is *not* deep-trance hypnosis. It is merely the *conscious* use of phrases and images which, through repetition, become subconscious implants. The effect of these implants is to relax the brain and help restore a normal balance between the sympathetic and parasympathetic divisions of the autonomic nervous system. Obviously, it is not designed to solve profound psychological problems. If such problems are known to exist or even suspected, professional help should be sought immediately.

**The role of nutrition**

There is one final point that must be made to round out the picture. Even though little has been written about the role of nutrition in the control of allergy, it stands to reason that this can be an important factor. If it is true that allergy involves a malfunction of the nervous system, then it is logical to do everything possible to strengthen that system. It is likely that the neurological stress threshold could be improved by rest, a well-rounded diet, avoidance of food additives and excess sugar commonly found in "junk foods," avoidance of needless neurological stimulants or depressants such as coffee, alcohol, or recreational drugs, and by the intake of certain supplements, particularly the vitamin B complex and trace minerals such as calcium, manganese, and potassium. All of these are known to be beneficial to neurological tissue, so their inclusion among the weaponry against allergy is strongly suggested.

This, then, is the picture. Allergy is a disease involving the chemical, mechanical, and neurological systems of the body. The controlling system, however, appears to be the neurological which is caused to malfunction by emotional stress. This malfunction throws the chemical and mechanical systems into turmoil resulting in the classical symptoms of allergy. If the cause of the malfunction is stress, assuming that in most cases the source of the stress cannot be removed, then the restoration of normalcy lies in helping the mind to *overcome* the stress by raising the neurological stress threshold.

**Summary**

This is the basis of The One-Ten-Ten Method.

There is nothing in this technique that is mutually exclusive to traditional methods. By its very nature, it is a non-drug approach to allergy control. Many patients, however, will continue to benefit from drug therapy and desensitization. The One-Ten-Ten Method can be used either as a supplement or alternative to such treatments. What we are proposing, however, is a slightly new perspective. In the past, there has been a tendency for the allergist and the psychotherapist to view their disciplines as, if not opposed, at least parallel and

**Compatible with traditional treatments**

separate. Here is a tool, however, that should be just as useful in the hands of one as in the other. It bridges the gap, so to speak, and, equally important, it makes it possible for the patient himself to participate in the resolution of his own disease.

It is an interesting comment upon our times that, in an era of billion-dollar research projects in all aspects of medicine and health, the most significant strides often are made, not by the medical giants funded by government or foundation grants, but by lone researchers paying their own expenses or by patients themselves who, in desperation, have been forced to experiment and to seek out alternatives.

It was just such desperation and experimentation that led to the development of The One-Ten-Ten Method. By sharing this discovery with his fellow allergy sufferers, John Laccinole has performed a service to mankind that is beyond measure. I am proud to be associated with his work.

It's dynamite!

**NOTES**     [1] Len J. Saul and James G. Delano, "Psychopathology and Psychotherapy in the Allergies of Children: A Review of the Literature," in *Somatic and Psychiatric Aspects of Childhood Allergies,* ed. Ernest Harms (New York: Pergamon, 1963), I, p. 2; see also G. F. Tucker, M.D., "Pulmonary Migraine," *Ann. Otol. Rhinol. Laryngol.,* 86 (1977), 671-76.

[2] Warren T. Vaughan, *Strange Malady: The Story of Allergy* (Garden City: Doubleday, 1941), pp. 220, 223, 225, 240.

[3] R.T. Long et al., "A Psychosomatic Study of Allergic and Emotional Factors in Children with Asthma," *Amer. J. Psychiat.,* 114 (1958), 890.

[4] Vaughan, p. 240.

[5] Vaughan, p. 236.

[6] Vaughan, p. 230.

[7] Vaughan, p. 230, 232.

[8] Harold Michal-Smith, "Psychological Aspects of the Allergic Child," in Harms, p. 62

[9] Vaughan, p. 237

[10] A. Tal and D.R. Miklich, "Emotionally Induced Decreases in Pulmonary Flow Rates in Asthmatic Children," *Psychosom. Med.,* 38 (1976), 190-200.

[11] K. Ezubalski and E. Rudzki, "Neuropsychic Factors in Physical Urticaria," *Dermatologica,* 154 (1977), 1-4

[12] P.G. Edgel, "Psychology of Asthma," *Canadian Med. Assn. I.,* 67 (1952), p. 121, cited in Michal-Smith, p. 52.

[13] B. Lask and D. Mathew, "Childhood Asthma: A Controlled Trial of Family Psychotherapy," *Arch. Dis. Child,* 54 (1979), 116-19.

[14] G. Schaeffer and H. Frytag-Klinger, "Objectifying the Effect of Autogenic Training on Disordered Ventilation in Bronchial Asthma," *Psychiatr. Neurol. Med. Psychol.,* 27 (1975), 400-08.

[15] Warren T. Vaughan and J. Harvey Black, *The Practice of Allergy* (St. Louis: C.V. Mosby, 1954), cited in Saul, p. 14.

[16] B. Ratner, ed., *Allergy in Relation to Pediatrics* (St. Paul: Bruce Publishing Co., 1951)

[17] Michal-Smith, p. 64

[18] R.M. Miller and R.W. Coger, "Skin Conductance Conditioning with Dyshidrotic Eczema Patients," *Br. J. Dermatology,* 101 (1979), 435-40.

[19] G.M. Aronoff, S. Aronoff, and L.W. Peck, "Hypnotherapy in the Treatment of Bronchial Asthma," *Ann. Allergy,* 34 (1975), 356-62.

[20] D.R. Collison, "Which Asthmatic Patients Should be Treated with Hypnotherapy?" *Med. J. Aust.,* 1 (1975), 776-81.

# A SUSPICIOUS PROFILE

by G. Edward Griffin    ©1980

*A review of the medical literature relating to an allergy personality profile: consideration of the effect that being chronically ill can have on personality traits; evidence that allergy victims have higher anxiety levels than those with other illnesses; measuring the difference between anxiety related to the illness and anxiety as part of a general life-pattern; involvement of the endocrine system; failure of behavior modification, relevancy of The One-Ten-Ten Method.*

In chapter three, Mr. Laccinole reviewed the emotional factors that were operative in his own life during his battle against allergy and suggested that they may be fairly representative of similar factors to be found in the lives of many other allergy sufferers. When I first read his manuscript I wondered if that could be substantiated, so I included it on the list of things to look for during my survey of the medical literature. Here is what I found.

**Much research
has been done**

First of all, I was surprised to discover that the question of an allergy personality profile has received an enormous amount of attention in research circles. While there is considerable difference of opinion regarding the exact form of that profile, there is little challenge to the *existence* of such a profile.

**The effect of
socio-psychological
factors**

Why is this important? Because it is the psychological aspect of the disease that determines the outcome of therapy, and the more we know about that aspect, the better chance we have of effecting a satisfactory cure. This question of the dominant importance of psychological factors cannot be over emphasized. For example, when a group of asthmatics who had become cured without any specific treatment was compared with a similar age group who still suffered from the disease, it was shown that the severity of the illness or the predisposition to it was not a factor. In other words, very severe cases were found in both groups equally, not just in the continuing asthma group. The study concluded: "These findings suggest that allergic predisposition does not influence the prognosis (chances of becoming cured) of allergic disorders as much as do socio-psychological factors."[1]

We are interested in the possibility of an allergy personality profile, therefore, because, if it exists, it could be one of the most important "socio-psychological factors" at work determining the potential success or failure of any therapy.

**A survey of cases**

Here is a survey of some of the studies that have explored this question. Little and Cohen reported that asthmatic children and their mothers set higher goals than others and that striving for these goals was a dominant factor in their lives.[2] Greenfield showed that victims of allergy displayed a higher than average need for recognition.[3] Alcock used the Rorschach test (interpreting ink blotches) and concluded that asthmatic children had high sensitivity in personal relationships, a high degree of tension without appropriate release, and inhibition in the use of their intelligence.[4] Nehans reported that asthmatic children had significantly higher levels of anxiety, insecurity, and dependence.[5] The significant aspect of this study was that heart patients were included in the test to see if some of the personality traits might be common to all children suffering from disease, a possible case of the condition of illness causing the personality trait rather than the trait causing the illness. The results, however, confirmed that the heart patients scored as average on most counts. Only the asthmatic children stood apart.

One of the more recent studies along this line is also one of the most complete. The work originally was published in the Scandinavian psychiatric journals. In it Dr. Sharma and Dr. Nandkumar report:

**Unrealistically high goals**

> The results revealed that the asthmatics were intelligent but inhibited. They had covert aggression, neurotic constriction, and marked affectional and dependency needs. They had considerable anxiety and were unable to use their energy for constructive work.... They were possessed with irrational fears, guilt feelings, and insecurity. Though high goals were set, they were unable to achieve them.[6]

In 1977, the sleep disorder unit at the Mount Sinai Medical Center in Miami Beach, Florida, released a study showing that nocturnal bruxism (tooth grinding) was three times more prevalent among children with allergies than among those without.[7] Although the purpose of the study was not to determine the reason for this tooth grinding in sleep, the report did point out that "psychogenic" factors could be involved.

**Tooth grinding in sleep**

As mentioned previously, there remains a gnawing suspicion that the commonly observed anxiety and depression traits could be indirect products of the allergy, not the cause of it. After all, who wouldn't be

**The chicken or the egg controversy**

anxious and depressed under the same circumstances? Fortunately, more recent experiments have taken this possibility into account. Instead of just one control group of people without allergies, they now are including a second control group composed of those who suffer from similar disabling diseases which logically should produce just about the same psychological pressure toward fear, frustration, and despair. This model was used by Dr. Ahmar and Dr. Kurban in a study of patients with allergic dermatitis. Patients with other kinds of dermatological disorders also were included, as were, of course, a group of persons with no symptoms of any kind. The results showed that those with allergic dermatitis and those with other skin disorders had different personality traits than normal individuals. This tends to support the supposition that the experience of having a skin disease can help to shape the personality of the patient. The important point, however, is that the two groups with skin disorders also scored significantly differently from each other.

The report concluded:

**The controversy is resolved**

> The study clearly shows that patients with atopic allergic dermatitis have a characteristic psychological profile not shared by the other two groups. The atopic dermatitis patients tend to be in a state of high manifest anxiety, depressed, neurotic, and hypochondriac.[8]

**Two kinds of anxiety**

Now we are really getting into something interesting. There are *two* kinds of anxiety. One is caused by the state of being ill and is referred to in the literature as *state anxiety*. The other is associated with the personality trait of the patient and, accordingly, is called *trait anxiety*. It is possible with proper testing techniques to measure each of them separately. When this is done, we find that high levels of anxiety related to the allergy itself (state) are relatively unimportant in the eventual outcome of the disease. It is the level of *trait* anxiety that makes the difference. The higher it is, the less likely are statistical chances of improvement or recovery.[9]

Why should this be so? Think back for a moment to our previous discussion of the autonomic nervous system and its subcomponents, the sympathetic and parasympathetic. We recall that the parasympathetic can be stimulated by the action of stress upon the hypothalamus and the pituitary. And that, in turn, cocks the trigger for an allergic reaction to the slightest environmental challenge. Stress, as measured by patient anxiety, therefore, is not just a *symptom* of allergy, it most probably is the *cause*. The higher the anxiety, the greater the cause.

**The effect of stress**

Everyone, of course, faces stress; some more than others, but over a lifetime most of us face enough situations with sufficient stress to produce an allergic reaction if we were inclined in that direction. The reason that some do and some don't has little to do with their intelligence, their courage, or their self-discipline. The reason that some handle stress differently than others could be merely a difference in their endocrine systems. Instead of it being all in their heads, it could well be all in their *glands!*

Dr. Warren Vaughan explains it this way:

> A unique feature of the sympathetic system is that it is connected directly with the adrenal glands, those little organs which manufacture adrenalin and deliver it directly into the blood. .... Adrenalin stimulates the cells to respond in the same way that they do for the sympathetic nerves, but the stimulation is many times more intense. It is the difference between clucking at a plodding horse and cracking a whip. When you get mad and "see red," as the saying goes,

**The role of the glands**

your adrenal glands have flooded the blood with adrenalin....

Stimulation of the parasympathetic causes the secretion of acetylcholine. This is a hormone comparable to adrenalin, but it is not secreted in such large amounts. In contrast with adrenalin, it is rapidly destroyed in the blood. As a consequence, it exerts its effect only in the neighborhood of the stimulation. There are certain regions where it seems to be especially abundant after stimulation, and these are our old familiar allergic shock tissues. If there is over activity of the parasympathetic system in the bronchi, acetylcholine is produced locally, the bronchial muscles go into spasm, and asthma results. Similar processes may occur in other shock tissues....

**Two types of people**

As far as the autonomic nervous system is concerned, there are two types of people: the adren-ergic and the cholin-ergic. The adren-ergic are those who secrete large amounts of adrenalin into the blood when they become excited. Their sympathetic systems are more active than the parasympathetics. They get mad and throw dishes. They are not the people who develop allergic symptoms. They adjust themselves explosively to environmental problems and have no further trouble.

The cholin-ergic crowd is controlled by their acetylcholine, by predominant activity of the parasympathetic system. They don't throw flatirons. They are reticent. They keep their problems to themselves. They do not "see red." Instead they break out with a crop of hives or have sick headaches.[10]

Does this mean that all one has to do to get rid of an

allergy is to set out to get steaming mad and start throwing dishes and flatirons? Not quite. Unfortunately, it's not that simple. This is not something for which you can train yourself. You either are that way or you aren't. Either you have an active adrenal system or you don't. Either you produce abundant acetylcholine or you don't. You may become angry, but if your acetylcholine production always accompanies or exceeds the production of adrenalin, your parasympathetic system still will be dominant.

**Losing one's temper is not enough**

This was illustrated quite graphically in a 1978 experiment in which a group of asthmatic children was given relaxation training, another group given assertiveness training, and a third group was given both. At the conclusion of the eight-week program, respiratory function was measured and compared to results obtained at the start of the program. The children who underwent relaxation training alone and those who combined relaxation training with assertiveness training showed an improved respiratory function. The children undergoing assertiveness training without relaxation training, however, had no improvement in respiratory function and actually were experiencing an *increase* in the frequency of attacks.[11] The lesson was clear. You can teach a child to be assertive, but if that is contrary to his basic nature, the new and uncomfortable behavior pattern may only add a new dimension of stress and anxiety that previously did not exist. It is possible, of course, that behavior modification applied over a sufficient length of time could, by some diverse mechanism, begin to alter the endocrine system itself. To date, however, there is no evidence to support such a view. So, you might just as well keep those dishes intact.

**The effect of assertiveness training**

It is commonly observed that children with an asthmatic parent, particularly the mother, are more apt to develop asthma themselves. Indications are that the correlation rates are as high as sixty per cent.[12] It is often assumed, therefore, that allergies in general and asthma

**The hereditary factor**

in particular are genetically inherited. If this is true, it is possible that the foci of genetic transmission lay in the endocrine system. Furthermore, the possibility also exists that emotional factors are transmitted from parent to child, not by genetic inheritance, but by the example of behavior. Add to this the third possibility that, since families tend to perpetuate the same eating habits, menus, and dietary patterns passed from grandmother to mother to daughter, a state of marginal nutritional deficiency also could play a role.

**Summary**    Add all of this together and it is easy to see that what is not known about the allergic personality profile is far greater than what is. There is considerable disagreement over the exact contour of that profile, but almost universal agreement that (1) it definitely exists and (2) the common denominator is anxiety. As to the *source* of that anxiety? Professional opinion varies considerably on this question and includes such diverse theories as mother rejection, traumatic toilet training, inhibited speech development, surpressed crying syndrome, rival siblings, goal striving, sexual repression, subconscious guilt, and behavior mimicing. Take your pick. For our purposes here, it is not necessary that we solve this puzzle. Whatever the cause or causes may be, the end result is anxiety. The beauty of The One-Ten-Ten Method is that it allows us to attack the anxiety syndrome directly. Naturally, it would be nice if it were possible to discover the specific cause of that anxiety for each individual and then go to work to eliminate it. But that is the special province of the psychotherapist. It should be emphasized again that, where serious personality patterns or deep-seated psychological conflicts are known to exist, or even if they are suspected, professional help should be sought immediately. The reality, however, is that, for most allergy sufferers, psychotherapy is both impractical and unnecessary. The cause of their anxieties will probably continue more or less throughout most of their lives. The objective of The One-Ten-Ten Method, therefore, is to help them live *with* those causes and to condition their nervous systems to function more normally in *spite* of the stress.

**NOTES**

[1] Y. Ago et al., "Psychosomatic Studies of Allergic Disorders," *Psychother. Psychosom.* 31 (1979), 197-204.

[2] S.W. Little and L.D. Cohen, "Goal Setting Behavior of Asthmatic Children and of Their Mothers for Them," *J. Person.,* 19 (1951), 376.

[3] N.S. Greenfield, "Allergy and the Need for Recognition," *J. Consulting Psychol.,* 22 (1958), 230-32.

[4] T. Alcock, "Some Personality Characteristics of Asthmatic Children," *Brit. J. Med. Psychol.,* 33 (1960), 133-41.

[5] E.C. Nehans, "A Personality Study of Asthmatic and Cardiac Children," *Psychosom. Med.,* 20 (1958), 181-86.

[6] S. Sharma and V.K. Nandkumar, "Personality Structure and Adjustment Pattern in Bronchial Asthma," *Acta. Psychiatr. Scand.,* 61 (1980), 81-88

[7] M.B. Marks, "Bruxism in Allergic Children," *Amer. J. Orthod.,* 77 (1980), 48-59

[8] H. Ahmar and A.K. Kurban, "Psychological Profile of Patients with Atopic Dermatitis," *Br. J. Dermatology,* 95 (1976), 373-77.

[9] J.F. Dirks et al., "Panic-Fear in Asthma: Symptomatology as an Index of Signal Anxiety and Personality as an Index of Ego Resources," *J. Nerv. Ment. Dis.,* 167 (1979), 615-19; J.F. Dirks, K.H. Fross, and N.W. Evans, "Panic-Fear in Asthma: Generalized Personality Trait *vs.* Specific Situation State," *J. Asthma Res.,* 14 (1977), 161-67.

[10] Warren T. Vaughan, *Strange Malady: The Story of Allergy* (Garden City: Doubleday, 1941), pp. 232-33, 237.

[11] R.A. Hocks et al.,"Medico-Psychological Interventions in Male Asthmatic Children: An Evaluation of Physiological Change," *Psychosom. Med.,* 40 (1978), 210-15.

[12] Jerome Glasser, "The Prophylaxis of Allergic Disease in Infancy and Childhood," in *Somatic and Psychiatric Aspects of Childhood Allergies,* ed. Ernest Harms (New York: Pergamon, 1963), I, 75.

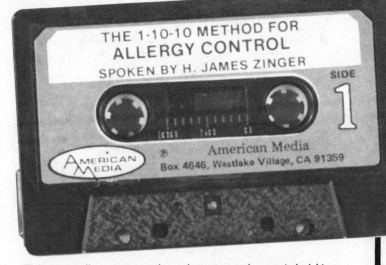

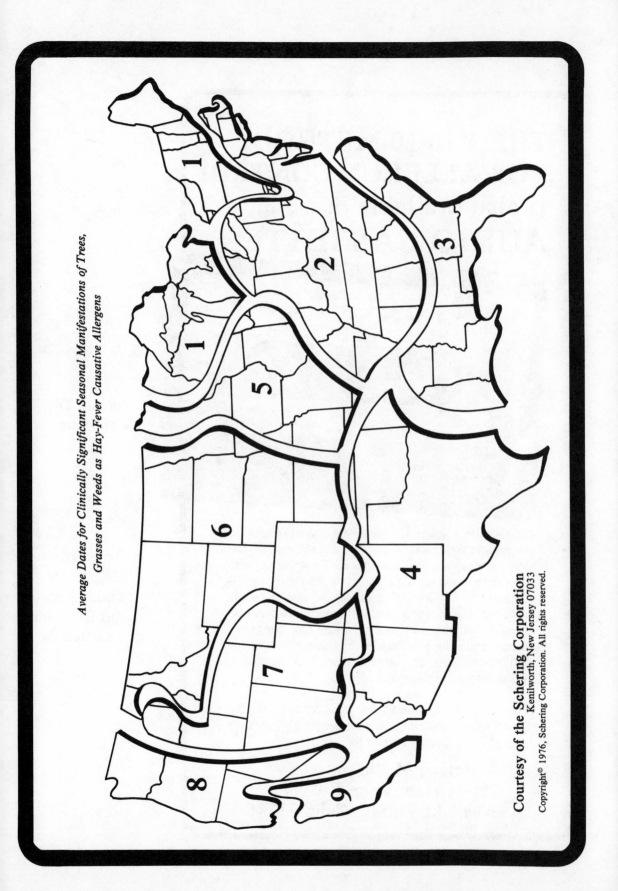

*Average Dates for Clinically Significant Seasonal Manifestations of Trees, Grasses and Weeds as Hay-Fever Causative Allergens*

**Courtesy of the Schering Corporation**
Kenilworth, New Jersey 07033

# ALLERGY ALERT!

## Are airborne pollens invading your area?

This map and chart identify major pollen sources and their prevalent time periods.

To determine when the most common airborne pollens will attack your area, look under the column heading with your zone number, on the chart below.

| COMMON AND SCIENTIFIC NAME | ZONE 1 | ZONE 2 | ZONE 3 | ZONE 4 | ZONE 5 | ZONE 6 | ZONE 7 | ZONE 8 | ZONE 9 |
|---|---|---|---|---|---|---|---|---|---|
| Poplar, Cottonwood: *Populus* | Apr-May | Apr | Mar-Apr | Mar-Apr | Mar-Apr | Mar-Apr-May | Apr-May | [1]Mar-Apr | Feb-Mar-Apr |
| Maple, Box elder: *Acer* | Apr-May | [1]Mar-Apr-May | Jan-Feb-Mar | Feb-Apr. inc. | Mar-Apr | Mar-Jun, inc. | Mar-Apr-May | Mar-Apr | Feb-Mar-Apr |
| Elm: *Ulmus* | Apr-May | Mar-Apr-May | Feb-Mar-Apr | Feb-Mar-Apr/Sept | Mar-Apr-May | Mar-Apr | Mar-Apr | Mar-Apr | |
| Oak: *Quercus* | May-Jun | [1]Apr-May | Jan-Feb-Mar-Apr | Mar-Apr-May | Apr-May | Apr-May | Apr-May | Mar-Apr | |
| Pecan, Hickory: *Carya* | Jun | May-Jun | Mar-Apr | Apr-Nov, inc. | May-Jun | | | | |
| Cedar, Juniper: *Juniperus* | Mar-Apr | May-Jun | Jan-Feb-Mar | [1]Jan-Apr/Nov-Dec | Mar-Apr | Mar-Apr-May | Apr | May | |
| Ash: *Fraxinus* | May-Jun | Apr-May | | [2]Mar-Apr/Sept | Apr-May | May | Apr-May | | |
| Walnut: *Juglans* | May-Jun | May | | Apr-May | May | | Apr-May | | Mar-Apr-May |
| Sycamore: *Platanus* | May-Jun | Apr-May | Jun | | | | | | Feb-Mar-Apr-May |
| Orchard grass: *Dactylis glomerata* | May-Jun | [1]May-Jun-Jul | Jun-Sept | | May-Jun-Jul | May-Jun-Jul | Jun-Jul | May-Jun-Jul | Apr-Aug, inc. |
| Timothy: *Phleum pratense* | Jun-Jul | May-Jun-Jul | Jun-Sept | | Jun-Jul | Jun-Jul | Jun-Jul | Jun-Jul-Aug | |
| June grass, Blue grasses: *Poa pratensis trivialis, annua* | May-Jun-Jul | [1]May-Jul, inc. | Mar-Apr/Jun | May-Aug, inc | May-Jun-Jul | May-Aug, inc. | May-Aug, inc. | May-Jun | [1]Apr-Aug, inc. |
| Sweet vernal grass: *Anthox. odor.* | May-Jun | May-Jun-Jul | | | Jun-Jul | | | May-Jun | |
| Bermuda grass: *Cynodon dactylon* | | [2]Jun-Jul-Aug-Sept | Apr-Sept, inc. | Apr-May-Jun/Oct | | Jun-Jul-Aug | Jun-Jul-Aug | Jun-Jul-Aug | [1]May-Oct, inc. |
| Redtop: *Agrostis alba* | May-Jun-Jul | Jun-Jul | May-Sept, inc. | Jul-Aug | Jun-Jul | Jun-Jul-Aug | Jun-Jul-Aug | Jun-Jul-Aug | Jun-Aug, inc. |
| Johnson grass, Sudan grass: *Holcus* | | Jun-Jul | May-Sept, inc. | Jun-Jul-Aug | Apr/Jul-Aug/Oct | Jun-Jul-Aug, inc. | May-Jul-Aug | May-Jul-Aug | Jun-Jul-Aug |
| Russian thistle: *Salsola pestifer* | [1]Aug | | | Jun-Jul-Aug | [1]Jul-Aug | Jul-Aug-Sept | Jul-Aug | Jul-Oct, inc. | Jun-Jul-Aug |
| Pigweed, Careless Weed, Tumbleweed: *Amaranthus* | Jun-Jul | Jun-Sept, inc. | Jun-Oct, inc. | [2]Jun-Sept, inc. | Jul-Aug-Sept | Jul-Oct, inc. | Jul-Aug | Jun-Sept, inc. | May-Sept, inc. |
| Saltbush, Shad scale: *Atriplex* | | | | [3]Jun-Sept, inc. | Jul-Aug | Jul-Aug-Sept | Jul-Aug-Sept | Jun-Sept, inc. | May-Sept, inc. |
| Western water hemp: *Acnida* | | [3]Jul-Aug-Sept | | [1]Jul-Aug-Sept | Jul-Aug | | | | |
| Lamb's-quarters: *Chenopodium album* | Jun-Jul | Jul-Aug-Sept | Aug-Sept-Oct | | Jun-Sept, inc. | Jun-Sept, inc. | Jul-Aug | Jul-Jul-Aug | |
| Wheat grass, Quack grass: *Agropyron* | Jun-Jul | | | Apr-Jul, inc. | Jul-Aug | Jun-Jul | May-Jun-Jul | Jun-Jul | |
| English plantain: *Plantago lanceolata* | May-Jun-Aug | May-Aug, inc. | Apr-May-Jun | May-Sept, inc. | Jun-Jul-Aug | Jun-Sept, inc. | May-Sept, inc. | May-Sept, inc. | May-Aug, inc. |
| Velvet grass: *Notholcus lanata* | | | | | | | | Jun-Jul | |
| Ray or Rye grass: *Lolium* | | May-Jun | May-Jun | Apr-May | Apr-Oct, inc | Jun-Jul | Jun-Jul-Aug | May-Aug, inc. | [1]May-Jun-Jul |
| Brome grass, Chess: *Bromus* | | May-Jun | Mar-Jun, inc. | Mar-May, inc. | Jun-Jul | Jun-Jul | Jun-Jul | May-Jul, inc. | Mar-Apr-May |
| Oat, wild and cultivated: *Avena* | | | Aug-Nov, inc. | | | | | Mar-Jun, inc. | |
| Marsh elder: *Iva* | | Aug-Sept | | Sept-Oct | [1]Aug-Sept | Jul-Aug-Sept | Jun-Sept, inc. | Aug-Sept | Jul-Aug-Sept |
| Sagebrush, Wormwood, Mugwort: *Artemisia* | Jul-Aug-Sept | Jul-Aug-Sept | | Aug-Sept-Oct | [2]Aug-Sept | Aug-Sept | Aug-Sept-Oct | Jun-Sept, inc. | Jun-Nov, inc. |
| Burning bush: *Kochia scoparia* | | | | Aug-Nov, inc. | Aug-Sept | [1]Jul-Aug-Sept | Jul-Aug | | [2]Jun-Oct, inc. |
| Giant ragweed: *Ambrosia trifida* | Aug-Sept | Aug-Sept | | [4]Aug-Sept-Oct | Aug-Sept | [1]Jul-Aug-Sept | | | |
| Dwarf ragweed: *Ambrosia elatior* | Aug-Sept | Aug-Sept | [1]Jul-Nov, inc. | [4]Aug-Nov, inc. | Aug-Sept | [1]Aug-Sept-Oct | Aug-Sept-Oct | [2]Aug-Sept-Oct | |
| Western ragweed: *Ambrosia psilostachya* | | | [2]Aug-Sept-Oct | [5]Aug-Oct, inc. | Aug-Sept | [1]Aug-Sept | Aug-Sept | [2]Aug-Sept-Oct | Jul-Aug-Sept |
| False ragweed: *Franseria* | | | | Mar-Apr-May | Jul-Aug-Sept | [1]Aug-Sept | Jul-Aug-Sept | [2]Apr-May/Aug-Sept | Jun-Oct, inc. |
| Pine: *Pinaceae* | | | Feb-Apr | | | | | May-Jun | |

**ZONE 1:** (1) Western portion of zone only.

**ZONE 2:** (1) Pollinates 1-2 mos. earlier in southern portion. (2) Occurs only in southern portion. (3) Occurs in western portion only.

**ZONE 3:** (1) Chiefly in western portion. None in Florida. (2) None in eastern Florida.

**ZONE 4:** (1) Less common in western portion. (2) Pollinates perennially in protected areas in eastern portion. (3) Less common in western portion. (4) None in western portion. (5) Pollinates earlier in extreme western Texas.

**ZONE 5:** (1) None in Milwaukee, Wis. (2) Little in Omaha, Neb., and Milwaukee. (3) Less common in Milwaukee.

**ZONE 6:** (1) None in western Colorado, western Montana, or northern Idaho.

**ZONE 8:** (1) Pollinates one month earlier in southern portion. (2) None in northern portion.

**ZONE 9:** (1) Pollinates perennially in certain areas, especially in southern portion. (2) Less common in southern portion.

# ALLERGY CASE RECORD
# AND WEEKLY
# PROGRESS RECORDS

The key to success with The One-Ten-Ten Method is perseverance. Those who utilize the program daily will become the winners who make it work. Those who only dabble with it once or twice a week are not likely to find relief. If you are really serious about solving your allergy problem, therefore, you must make up your mind now to place this item at the very top of your list of priorities.

To help you get started, you will find on the following pages one case record and thirteen weekly progress records. Their purpose is:
(1) To prompt you to a more faithful adherence to the daily exercises. Most of us do better when we have a track to run on.
(2) To provide a convenient way to monitor your own progress.

Daily entries should be made throughout the entire thirteen week period or until you feel that your allergy is under control, should that occur in less than thirteen weeks. Complete the bottom half of the case record only when you terminate your record-keeping for one of these two reasons.

# ALLERGY CASE RECORD

**(Please complete this section at the start of the 1-10-10 Method)**

| | |
|---|---|
| NAME: | |
| ADDRESS: | |
| | ZIP: |

| AGE WHEN SYMPTOMS FIRST APPEARED: | AGE AT START OF METHOD: | DATE AT START OF METHOD: |
|---|---|---|

SYMPTOMS:

PRIOR TREATMENTS: AND RESULTS:

**(Please complete this section at the conclusion of your record-keeping)**

| DATE AT END OF RECORD-KEEPING: | NO. OF WEEKLY CHARTS COMPLETED: | TOTAL TIMES METHOD WAS APPLIED: |
|---|---|---|
| METHOD WAS APPLIED: | ☐ OUT LOUD        ☐ SILENT | ☐ FROM AUDIO CASSETTE |
| METHOD WAS USED: | ☐ WITHOUT DRUGS    ☐ WITH REDUCED DRUG THERAPY | ☐ WITH THE SAME THERAPY USED BEFORE |
| RESULTS AT END OF RECORD-KEEPING: | ☐ EXCELLENT    ☐ GOOD    ☐ FAIR | ☐ POOR |

OBSERVATIONS AND COMMENTS:

## WEEK NUMBER 1

| DAY | NO. OF TIMES METHOD WAS REPEATED THIS DAY | RESULTS AT END OF DAY (CHECK ONE) | | | |
|---|---|---|---|---|---|
| | | EXCELLENT | GOOD | FAIR | POOR |
| MONDAY | | | | | |
| TUESDAY | | | | | |
| WEDNESDAY | | | | | |
| THURSDAY | | | | | |
| FRIDAY | | | | | |
| SATURDAY | | | | | |
| SUNDAY | | | | | |
| OBSERVATIONS AND COMMENTS: | | | | | |

## WEEK NUMBER 2

| DAY | NO. OF TIMES METHOD WAS REPEATED THIS DAY | RESULTS AT END OF DAY (CHECK ONE) | | | |
|---|---|---|---|---|---|
| | | EXCELLENT | GOOD | FAIR | POOR |
| MONDAY | | | | | |
| TUESDAY | | | | | |
| WEDNESDAY | | | | | |
| THURSDAY | | | | | |
| FRIDAY | | | | | |
| SATURDAY | | | | | |
| SUNDAY | | | | | |
| OBSERVATIONS AND COMMENTS: | | | | | |

## WEEK NUMBER 3

| DAY | NO. OF TIMES METHOD WAS REPEATED THIS DAY | RESULTS AT END OF DAY (CHECK ONE) | | | |
|---|---|---|---|---|---|
| | | EXCELLENT | GOOD | FAIR | POOR |
| MONDAY | | | | | |
| TUESDAY | | | | | |
| WEDNESDAY | | | | | |
| THURSDAY | | | | | |
| FRIDAY | | | | | |
| SATURDAY | | | | | |
| SUNDAY | | | | | |
| OBSERVATIONS AND COMMENTS: | | | | | |

## WEEK NUMBER 4

| DAY | NO. OF TIMES METHOD WAS REPEATED THIS DAY | RESULTS AT END OF DAY (CHECK ONE) | | | |
|---|---|---|---|---|---|
| | | EXCELLENT | GOOD | FAIR | POOR |
| MONDAY | | | | | |
| TUESDAY | | | | | |
| WEDNESDAY | | | | | |
| THURSDAY | | | | | |
| FRIDAY | | | | | |
| SATURDAY | | | | | |
| SUNDAY | | | | | |
| OBSERVATIONS AND COMMENTS: | | | | | |

## WEEK NUMBER 5

| DAY | NO. OF TIMES METHOD WAS REPEATED THIS DAY | RESULTS AT END OF DAY (CHECK ONE) | | | |
|---|---|---|---|---|---|
| | | EXCELLENT | GOOD | FAIR | POOR |
| MONDAY | | | | | |
| TUESDAY | | | | | |
| WEDNESDAY | | | | | |
| THURSDAY | | | | | |
| FRIDAY | | | | | |
| SATURDAY | | | | | |
| SUNDAY | | | | | |
| OBSERVATIONS AND COMMENTS: | | | | | |
| | | | | | |
| | | | | | |
| | | | | | |

## WEEK NUMBER 6

| DAY | NO. OF TIMES METHOD WAS REPEATED THIS DAY | RESULTS AT END OF DAY (CHECK ONE) | | | |
|---|---|---|---|---|---|
| | | EXCELLENT | GOOD | FAIR | POOR |
| MONDAY | | | | | |
| TUESDAY | | | | | |
| WEDNESDAY | | | | | |
| THURSDAY | | | | | |
| FRIDAY | | | | | |
| SATURDAY | | | | | |
| SUNDAY | | | | | |
| OBSERVATIONS AND COMMENTS: | | | | | |
| | | | | | |
| | | | | | |
| | | | | | |

## WEEK NUMBER 7

| DAY | NO. OF TIMES METHOD WAS REPEATED THIS DAY | RESULTS AT END OF DAY (CHECK ONE) | | | |
|---|---|---|---|---|---|
| | | EXCELLENT | GOOD | FAIR | POOR |
| MONDAY | | | | | |
| TUESDAY | | | | | |
| WEDNESDAY | | | | | |
| THURSDAY | | | | | |
| FRIDAY | | | | | |
| SATURDAY | | | | | |
| SUNDAY | | | | | |
| OBSERVATIONS AND COMMENTS: | | | | | |
| | | | | | |
| | | | | | |
| | | | | | |

## WEEK NUMBER 8

| DAY | NO. OF TIMES METHOD WAS REPEATED THIS DAY | RESULTS AT END OF DAY (CHECK ONE) | | | |
|---|---|---|---|---|---|
| | | EXCELLENT | GOOD | FAIR | POOR |
| MONDAY | | | | | |
| TUESDAY | | | | | |
| WEDNESDAY | | | | | |
| THURSDAY | | | | | |
| FRIDAY | | | | | |
| SATURDAY | | | | | |
| SUNDAY | | | | | |
| OBSERVATIONS AND COMMENTS: | | | | | |
| | | | | | |
| | | | | | |
| | | | | | |

## WEEK NUMBER 9

| DAY | NO. OF TIMES METHOD WAS REPEATED THIS DAY | RESULTS AT END OF DAY (CHECK ONE) | | | |
|-----|-------------------------------------------|-----------|------|------|------|
|     |                                           | EXCELLENT | GOOD | FAIR | POOR |
| MONDAY | | | | | |
| TUESDAY | | | | | |
| WEDNESDAY | | | | | |
| THURSDAY | | | | | |
| FRIDAY | | | | | |
| SATURDAY | | | | | |
| SUNDAY | | | | | |
| OBSERVATIONS AND COMMENTS: | | | | | |

## WEEK NUMBER 10

| DAY | NO. OF TIMES METHOD WAS REPEATED THIS DAY | RESULTS AT END OF DAY (CHECK ONE) | | | |
|-----|-------------------------------------------|-----------|------|------|------|
|     |                                           | EXCELLENT | GOOD | FAIR | POOR |
| MONDAY | | | | | |
| TUESDAY | | | | | |
| WEDNESDAY | | | | | |
| THURSDAY | | | | | |
| FRIDAY | | | | | |
| SATURDAY | | | | | |
| SUNDAY | | | | | |
| OBSERVATIONS AND COMMENTS: | | | | | |

## WEEK NUMBER 11

| DAY | NO. OF TIMES METHOD WAS REPEATED THIS DAY | RESULTS AT END OF DAY (CHECK ONE) | | | |
|---|---|---|---|---|---|
| | | EXCELLENT | GOOD | FAIR | POOR |
| MONDAY | | | | | |
| TUESDAY | | | | | |
| WEDNESDAY | | | | | |
| THURSDAY | | | | | |
| FRIDAY | | | | | |
| SATURDAY | | | | | |
| SUNDAY | | | | | |
| OBSERVATIONS AND COMMENTS: | | | | | |

## WEEK NUMBER 12

| DAY | NO. OF TIMES METHOD WAS REPEATED THIS DAY | RESULTS AT END OF DAY (CHECK ONE) | | | |
|---|---|---|---|---|---|
| | | EXCELLENT | GOOD | FAIR | POOR |
| MONDAY | | | | | |
| TUESDAY | | | | | |
| WEDNESDAY | | | | | |
| THURSDAY | | | | | |
| FRIDAY | | | | | |
| SATURDAY | | | | | |
| SUNDAY | | | | | |
| OBSERVATIONS AND COMMENTS: | | | | | |

## WEEK NUMBER 13

| DAY | NO. OF TIMES METHOD WAS REPEATED THIS DAY | RESULTS AT END OF DAY (CHECK ONE) | | | |
|---|---|---|---|---|---|
| | | EXCELLENT | GOOD | FAIR | POOR |
| MONDAY | | | | | |
| TUESDAY | | | | | |
| WEDNESDAY | | | | | |
| THURSDAY | | | | | |
| FRIDAY | | | | | |
| SATURDAY | | | | | |
| SUNDAY | | | | | |
| OBSERVATIONS AND COMMENTS: | | | | | |
| | | | | | |
| | | | | | |
| | | | | | |

# BIBLIOGRAPY

Ago, Y., et al. "Psychosomatic Studies of Allergic Disorders." *Psychother. Psychosom.,* 31 (1979), 197-204.

Ahmar, H., and A.K. Kurban, "Psychological Profile of Patients with Atopic Dermatitis." *Br. J. Dermatology,* 95 (1976), 373-77.

Alcock, T. "Some Personality Characteristics of Asthmatic Children. *Brit. J. Med. Psychol.,* 33 (1960), 133-41.
"Allergy." *Colliers Encyclopedia.* 1959 ed.
"Allergy and Anaphylaxis." *Encyclopedia Britannica.* 1964 ed.

Arnoff, G.M., S. Arnoff, and L.W. Peck. "Hypnotherapy in the Treatment of Bronchial Asthma." *Ann. Allergy,* 34 (1975), 356-62.

Collison, D.R. "Which Asthmatic Patients Should be Treated with Hypnotherapy?" *Med. J. Aust.,* 1 (1975), 776-81.

Dirks, J.F., et al. "Panic-Fear in Asthma: Symptomatology as an Index of Signal Anxiety and Personality as an Index of Ego Resources." *J. Nerv. Ment. Dis.,* 167 (1979), 615-19.

Dirks, J.F., K.H. Fross, and N.W. Evans. "Panic-Fear in Asthma: Generalized Personality Trait vs. Specific Situation State." *J. Asthma Res.,* 14 (1977), 161-67.

Edgel, P.G. "Psychology of Asthma." *Canadian Med. Assn.,* I. 67 (1952), p. 121.

Ezubolski, K., and E. Rudzki. "Neuropsychic Factors in Physical Urticaria." *Dermatologica,* 154 (1977) 1-4.

Gerrard,John W. *Understanding Allergies.* Springfield: Thomas Books, 1973.

Glaser, Jerome. "The Prophylaxis of Allergic Disease in Infancy and Childhood." in *Somatic and Psychiatric Aspects of Childhood Allergies.* Ed. Ernest Harms. New York: Pergamon, 1963, I, p. 75.

Greenfield, N.S. "Allergy and the Need for Recognition." *J. Consulting Psychol.,* 22 (1958), 230-32.

Harms, Ernest, ed. *Somatic and Psychiatric Aspects of Childhood Allergies.* New York: Pergamon, 1963.

Harris, M. Coleman, and Norman Shure. *All About Allergy.* Englewood Cliffs: Prentice Hall, 1969.

"Hay Fever." *Colliers Encyclopedia.* 1959 ed.

Hocks, R.A., et al. "Medico-Psychological Interventions in Male Asthmatic Children: An Evaluation of Physiological Change." *Psychosom. Med.,* 40 (1978), 210-15.

Lask, B., and D. Mathew. "Childhood Asthma: A Controlled Trial of Family Psychotherapy." *Arch. Dis. Child,* 54 (1979), 116-19.

Little, S.W., and L.D. Cohen. "Goal Setting Behavior of Asthmatic Children and of Their Mothers for Them." *J. Person.,* 19 (1951), 376.

Long, R.T., et al. "A Psychosomatic Study of Allergic and Emotional Factors in Children with Asthma." *Amer. J. Psychiat.,* 114 (1958), 890.

Marks, M.B. "Bruxism in Allergic Children." *Amer. J. Orthod.,* 77 (1980), 48-59.

Michal-Smith, Harold. "Psychological Aspects of the Allergic Child." in *Somatic and Psychiatric Aspects of Childhood Allergies.* Ed. Ernest Harms. New York: Pergamon, 1963, I, pp. 62, 64.

Miller, R.M., and R.W. Coger. "Skin Conductance Conditioning with Dyshidrotic Eczema Patients." *Br. J. Dermatology, 101 (1979), 435-40.*

Nehans, E.C. "A Personality Study of Asthmatic and Cardiac Children." *Psychosom. Med.,* 20 (1958), 181-86.

Ratner, B., ed. *Allergy in Relation to Pediatrics.* St. Paul: Bruce Publishing Co., 1951.

Saul, Len J., and James G. Delano. "Psychopathology and Psychotherapy in the Allergies of Children: A Review of the Literature." in *Somatic and Psychiatric Aspects of Childhood Allergies.* Ed. Ernest Harms. New York: Pergamon, 1963, I, p. 2.

Schaeffer, G., and H. Fryta-Klinger. "Objectifying the Effect of Autogenic Training on Disordered Ventilation in Bronchial Asthma." *Psychiatr. Neurol. Med. Psychol.,* 27 (1975), 400-08.

Sharma, S., and V.K. Nandkumar. "Personality Structure and Adjustment Pattern in Bronchial Asthma." *Acta. Psychiatr. Scand.,* 61 (1980), 81-88.

Tal, A., and D.R. Miklich. "Emotionally Induced Decreases in Pulmonary Flow Rates in Asthmatic Children." *Psychosom. Med.,* 38 (1976), 190-200.

Tucker, G.F. "Pulmonary Migraine." *Ann. Otol. Rhinol. Laryngol.,* 86 (1977), 671-76.

Vaughan, Warren T. *Strange Malady: The Story of Allergy.* Garden City: Doubleday, 1941.

# INDEX